Male Urethral Reconstruction and the Management of Urethral Stricture Disease

Editor

LEE C. ZHAO

UROLOGIC CLINICS
OF NORTH AMERICA

www.urologic.theclinics.com

Consulting Editor
SAMIR S. TANEJA

February 2017 • Volume 44 • Number 1

ELSEVIER

1600 John F. Kennedy Boulevard ● Suite 1800 ● Philadelphia, Pennsylvania, 19103-2899

http://www.theclinics.com

UROLOGIC CLINICS OF NORTH AMERICA Volume 44, Number 1
February 2017 ISSN 0094-0143, ISBN-13: 978-0-323-49681-0

Editor: Kerry Holland
Developmental Editor: Alison Swety

Urologic Clinics of North America (ISSN 0094-0143) is published quarterly by Elsevier Inc., 360 Park Avenue South, New York, NY 10010-1710. Months of issue are February, May, August, and November. Business and Editorial Offices: 1600 John F. Kennedy Blvd., Suite 1800, Philadelphia, PA 19103-2899. Periodicals postage paid at New York, NY and additional mailing offices. Subscription prices are $360.00 per year (US individuals), $680.00 per year (US institutions), $100.00 per year (US students and residents), $415.00 per year (Canadian individuals), $850.00 per year (Canadian institutions), $515.00 per year (foreign individuals), $850.00 per year (foreign institutions), and $240.00 per year (Canadian and foreign students/residents). Foreign air speed delivery is included in all *Clinics* subscription prices. All prices are subject to change without notice. **POSTMASTER:** Send address changes to *Urologic Clinics of North America*, Elsevier Health Sciences Division, Subscription Customer Service, 3251 Riverport Lane, Maryland Heights, MO 63043. **Customer Service: 1-800-654-2452 (US). From outside the United States, call 1-314-447-8871. Fax: 1-314-447-8029. E-mail: JournalsCustomerServiceusa@elsevier.com (for print support)** and **JournalsOnlineSupport-usa@elsevier.com (for online support)**.

Reprints. For copies of 100 or more, of articles in this publication, please contact the Commercial Reprints Department, Elsevier Inc., 360 Park Avenue South, New York, New York 10010-1710. Tel.: 212-633-3874; Fax: 212-633-3820; E-mail: reprints@elsevier.com.

Urologic Clinics of North America is covered in MEDLINE/PubMed (*Index Medicus*), *Excerpta Medica, Current Contents/Clinical Medicine, Science Citation Index,* and *ISI/BIOMED.*

PROGRAM OBJECTIVE

The goal of *Urologic Clinics of North America* is to keep practicing urologists and urology residents up to date with current clinical practice in urology by providing timely articles reviewing the state of the art in patient care.

TARGET AUDIENCE

Practicing urologists, urology residents and other health care professionals practicing in the discipline of urology.

LEARNING OBJECTIVES

Upon completion of this activity, participants will be able to:

1. Review cost-effective and successful treatment strategies for urethral stricture disease.
2. Discuss alternative management strategies for urethral stricture disease.
3. Recognize possible side-effects and follow up following urethral stricture treatment.

ACCREDITATION

The Elsevier Office of Continuing Medical Education (EOCME) is accredited by the Accreditation Council for Continuing Medical Education (ACCME) to provide continuing medical education for physicians.

The EOCME designates this enduring material for a maximum of 15 *AMA PRA Category 1 Credit*(s)™. Physicians should claim only the credit commensurate with the extent of their participation in the activity.

All other health care professionals requesting continuing education credit for this enduring material will be issued a certificate of participation.

DISCLOSURE OF CONFLICTS OF INTEREST

The EOCME assesses conflict of interest with its instructors, faculty, planners, and other individuals who are in a position to control the content of CME activities. All relevant conflicts of interest that are identified are thoroughly vetted by EOCME for fair balance, scientific objectivity, and patient care recommendations. EOCME is committed to providing its learners with CME activities that promote improvements or quality in healthcare and not a specific proprietary business or a commercial interest.

The planning committee, staff, authors and editors listed below have identified no financial relationships or relationships to products or devices they or their spouse/life partner have with commercial interest related to the content of this CME activity:

Daniela Andrich, MD, MSc, FRCS; Benjamin N. Breyer, MD, MAS, FACS; Brendan Michael Browne, MD, MS; Jill C. Buckley, MD, FACS; Simon Bugeja, MD, MRCS (Ed), FEBU, MSC (Urol); Nicol C. Bush, MD; Brittney H. Cotta, MD; Prem Nath Dogra, MCh, DSc (Hon); Sean P. Elliott, MD, MS; Bradley A Erickson, MD, MS; Anjali Fortna; Anastasia Frost, MSc (Urol), MBChB; George M. Ghareeb, MD, MBA; Michael A. Granieri, MD; Judith C. Hagedorn, MD, MHS; Catherine R. Harris, MD; Matthias D. Hofer, MD; Kerry Holland; James N. Hotaling, MD, MS; Stella Ivaz, MBBS, BMus (Hons), MA, MRCS, FRCS (Urol); Pankaj M. Joshi, MD; Jyotsna Kulkarni, FRCS; Sanjay Kulkarni, MD; Indu Kumari; Sarah M. Lenherr, MD, MS; Jamie P. Levine, MD; Mya E. Levy, MD; Joceline S. Liu, MD; Ramiro J. Madden-Fuentes, MD; Allen F. Morey, MD; Anthony R. Mundy, PhD (Hon), MS, FRCP, FRCS, FRACS (Hon); Gregory Murphy, MD; Jeremy B. Myers, MD, FACS; Rishi Nayyar, MCh; Dmitriy Nikolavsky, MD; E. Charles Osterberg, MD; Andrew C. Peterson, MD; Prabhjot Singh, MCh; Warren T. Snodgrass, MD; Megan Suermann; Sandesh Surana, MD; Alison Swety; Alex J. Vanni, MD, FACS; Bryan B. Voelzke, MD, MS; Siddharth Yadav, MS; Yuka Yamaguchi, MD; Lee C. Zhao, MD, MS.

The planning committee, staff, authors and editors listed below have identified financial relationships or relationships to products or devices they or their spouse/life partner have with commercial interest related to the content of this CME activity:

William O. Brant, MD, FACS is a consultant/advisor for, with research support from, Boston Scientific Corporation.
Samir S. Taneja, MD is a consultant/advisor for Bayer HealthCare Pharmaceuticals, Eigen Pharma LLC, GTx, Inc., HealthTronics, Inc. and Hitachi, Ltd.

UNAPPROVED/OFF-LABEL USE DISCLOSURE

The EOCME requires CME faculty to disclose to the participants:

1. When products or procedures being discussed are off-label, unlabelled, experimental, and/or investigational (not US Food and Drug Administration [FDA] approved); and
2. Any limitations on the information presented, such as data that are preliminary or that represent ongoing research, interim analyses, and/or unsupported opinions. Faculty may discuss information about pharmaceutical agents that is outside of FDA-approved labelling. This information is intended solely for CME and is not intended to promote off-label use of these medications. If you have any questions, contact the medical affairs department of the manufacturer for the most recent prescribing information.

TO ENROLL

To enroll in the *Urologic Clinics of North America* Continuing Medical Education program, call customer service at 1-800-654-2452 or sign up online at http://www.theclinics.com/home/cme. The CME program is available to subscribers for an additional annual fee of USD $270.

METHOD OF PARTICIPATION

In order to claim credit, participants must complete the following:

1. Complete enrolment as indicated above.
2. Read the activity.
3. Complete the CME Test and Evaluation. Participants must achieve a score of 70% on the test. All CME Tests and Evaluations must be completed online.

CME INQUIRIES/SPECIAL NEEDS

For all CME inquiries or special needs, please contact elsevierCME@elsevier.com.

Contributors

CONSULTING EDITOR

SAMIR S. TANEJA, MD
The James M. Neissa and Janet Riha Neissa
Professor of Urologic Oncology; Professor of
Urology and Radiology; Director, Division of
Urologic Oncology; Co-Director, Department
of Urology, Smilow Comprehensive Prostate
Cancer Center, NYU Langone Medical Center,
New York, New York

EDITOR

LEE C. ZHAO, MD, MS
Assistant Professor, Department of Urology,
NYU Langone Medical Center, New York
University School of Medicine, New York,
New York

AUTHORS

DANIELA ANDRICH, MD, MSc, FRCS
Consultant Reconstructive Urologist, Institute
of Urology at UCLH, London, United Kingdom

WILLIAM O. BRANT, MD, FACS
Associate Professor, Genitourinary Injury and
Reconstructive Urology, Department of
Surgery, University of Utah, Salt Lake City,
Utah

BENJAMIN N. BREYER, MD, MAS, FACS
Department of Urology, University of California,
San Francisco, San Francisco, California

BRENDAN MICHAEL BROWNE, MD, MS
Department of Urology, Lahey Hospital and
Medical Center, Burlington, Massachusetts

JILL C. BUCKLEY, MD, FACS
Department of Urology, UC San Diego Health
System, San Diego, California

**SIMON BUGEJA, MD, MRCS (Ed), FEBU,
MSC (Urol)**
Fellow in Reconstructive Urology, Institute of
Urology at UCLH, London, United Kingdom

NICOL C. BUSH, MD
PARC Urology, Frisco, Texas

BRITTNEY H. COTTA, MD
Department of Urology, UC San Diego Health
System, San Diego, California

PREM NATH DOGRA, MCh, DSc (Hon)
Professor and Head, Department of Urology,
All India Institute of Medical Sciences,
New Delhi, India

SEAN P. ELLIOTT, MD, MS
Department of Urology, University of
Minnesota, Minneapolis, Minnesota

BRADLEY A. ERICKSON, MD, MS
Department of Urology, University of Iowa
Hospitals & Clinics, Iowa City, Iowa

ANASTASIA FROST, MSc (Urol), MBChB
Fellow in Reconstructive Urology, Institute of
Urology at UCLH, London, United Kingdom

GEORGE M. GHAREEB, MD, MBA
Department of Urology, University of Iowa
Hospitals & Clinics, Iowa City, Iowa

MICHAEL A. GRANIERI, MD
Division of Urology, Department of Surgery,
Duke University Medical Center, Durham,
North Carolina

JUDITH C. HAGEDORN, MD, MHS
Assistant Professor, Department of Urology,
University of Washington, Seattle, Washington

CATHERINE R. HARRIS, MD
Department of Urology, University of California,
San Francisco, San Francisco, California;
Department of Urology, Stanford University,
Palo Alto, California

MATTHIAS D. HOFER, MD
Department of Urology, University of Texas
Southwestern, Dallas, Texas

JAMES N. HOTALING, MD, MS
Assistant Professor, Genitourinary Injury and
Reconstructive Urology, Department of
Surgery, University of Utah, Salt Lake City,
Utah

**STELLA IVAZ, MBBS, BMus (Hons), MA,
MRCS, FRCS (Urol)**
Fellow in Reconstructive Urology, Institute of
Urology at UCLH, London, United Kingdom

PANKAJ M. JOSHI, MD
Kulkarni Reconstructive Urology Center, Pune,
India

JYOTSNA KULKARNI, FRCS
Kulkarni Reconstructive Urology Center, Pune,
India

SANJAY KULKARNI, MD
Kulkarni Reconstructive Urology Center, Pune,
India

SARA M. LENHERR, MD, MS
Assistant Professor, Genitourinary Injury and
Reconstructive Urology, Department of
Surgery, University of Utah, Salt Lake City,
Utah

JAMIE P. LEVINE, MD
Associate Professor of Plastic Surgery,
Hansjörg Wyss Department of Plastic Surgery,
New York University School of Medicine, New
York, New York

MYA E. LEVY, MD
Department of Urology, University of
Minnesota, Minneapolis, Minnesota

JOCELINE S. LIU, MD
Department of Urology, Feinberg School of
Medicine, Northwestern University, Chicago,
Illinois

RAMIRO J. MADDEN-FUENTES, MD
Division of Urology, Department of Surgery,
Duke University Medical Center, Durham,
North Carolina

ALLEN F. MOREY, MD
Department of Urology, University of Texas
Southwestern, Dallas, Texas

**ANTHONY R. MUNDY, PhD (Hon), MS,
FRCP, FRCS, FRACS (Hon)**
Professor of Urology, Institute of Urology at
UCLH, UCLH NHS Foundation Trust, Trust
Headquarters, London, United Kingdom

GREGORY MURPHY, MD
Department of Urology, University of California,
San Francisco, San Francisco, California

JEREMY B. MYERS, MD, FACS
Associate Professor, Genitourinary Injury and
Reconstructive Urology, Department of
Surgery, University of Utah, Salt Lake City,
Utah

RISHI NAYYAR, MCh
Assistant Professor, Department of Urology, All
India Institute of Medical Sciences, New Delhi,
India

DMITRIY NIKOLAVSKY, MD
Assistant Professor of Urology, Department of
Urology, Upstate University Hospital, SUNY
Upstate Medical University, Syracuse,
New York

E. CHARLES OSTERBERG, MD
Department of Urology, University of California,
San Francisco, San Francisco, California

ANDREW C. PETERSON, MD
Professor of Surgery, Division of Urology,
Department of Surgery, Duke University
Medical Center, Durham, North Carolina

PRABHJOT SINGH, MCh
Assistant Professor, Department of Urology, All
India Institute of Medical Sciences, New Delhi,
India

WARREN T. SNODGRASS, MD
PARC Urology, Frisco, Texas

SANDESH SURANA, MD
Kulkarni Reconstructive Urology Center, Pune, India

ALEX J. VANNI, MD, FACS
Department of Urology, Lahey Hospital and Medical Center, Burlington, Massachusetts

BRYAN B. VOELZKE, MD, MS
Associate Professor, Department of Urology, University of Washington, Seattle, Washington

SIDDHARTH YADAV, MS
Senior Resident, Department of Urology, All India Institute of Medical Sciences, New Delhi, India

YUKA YAMAGUCHI, MD
Attending Physician, Division of Urology, Department of Surgery, Highland Hospital, Alameda Health System, Oakland, California

LEE C. ZHAO, MD, MS
Assistant Professor, Department of Urology, NYU Langone Medical Center, New York University School of Medicine, New York, New York

Contents

In recent years, the issues of the transgender population have become more visible in the media worldwide. Transgender patients at various stages of their transformation will present to urologic clinics requiring general or specialized urologic care. Knowledge of specifics of reconstructed anatomy and potential unique complications of the reconstruction will become important in providing urologic care to these patients. In this article, we have concentrated on describing diagnosis and treatment of the more common urologic complications after female-to-male reconstructions: urethrocutaneous fistulae, neourethral strictures, and symptomatic persistent vaginal cavities.

The current management for complex urethral strictures commonly uses open reconstruction with buccal mucosa urethroplasty. However, there are multiple situations whereby buccal mucosa is inadequate (eg, pan-urethral stricture or prior buccal harvest) or inappropriate for utilization (eg, heavy tobacco use or oral radiation). Multiple options exist for use as alternatives or adjuncts to buccal mucosa in complex urethral strictures. This article reviews the current state of alternate techniques for urethral stricture treatment besides buccal mucosa, including injectable antifibrotic agents, augmentation urethroplasty with skin flaps, lingual mucosa, colonic mucosa, and new developments in tissue engineering for urethral graft material.

UROLOGIC CLINICS OF NORTH AMERICA

Preface
Management of Urethral Strictures

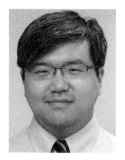

Lee C. Zhao, MD, MS
Editor

The management of urethral stricture has been revolutionized in the past 20 years with the popularization of buccal mucosa graft for adult urethroplasty, and now, most strictures of the urethra can be treated surgically with good outcomes. Despite evidence that repeat endoscopic treatment is less effective than urethroplasty, there remain many stricture patients who suffer through repeated futile endoscopic interventions and are never offered urethroplasty. Only education can change this dismal practice. As Guest Editor of this issue of *Urologic Clinics*, I aimed to provide an overview of the contemporary management of urethral stricture disease.

Standardized definitions of success are important for evaluation of surgical technique: we can only improve what we measure. This issue of *Urologic Clinics* begins with a declaration on how to define successful surgery, and the standardized follow-up after urethral reconstruction. The ideal follow-up regimen must be weighed against the cost, and the next article provides a discussion of cost-effectiveness.

Progress in the treatment of urethral strictures involves making surgery less morbid and more efficacious. Although less efficacious, endoscopy is the least morbid treatment and is often the preferred initial step of therapy. If urethroplasty is chosen, one must select between anastomotic and substitution urethroplasty, and for substitution urethroplasty, which grafts to use. Sexual dysfunction after urethroplasty can be a significant source of patient dissatisfaction. One surgical innovation

to reduce the risk of sexual dysfunction is the approach of nontransecting urethroplasty.

There are several challenging problems in urethral reconstruction that warrant detailed discussion. Panurethral strictures, lichen sclerosis, and radiation-induced strictures can all reduce the success rate of reconstruction. Another complicated topic is the management of urinary incontinence in patients with urethral strictures, as artificial urinary sphincter placement may result in urethral erosions, and urethral strictures may arise after urethral erosions. A detailed understanding of the reasons for failure of initial reconstruction is important for urethroplasty after complications of hypospadias surgery and for strictures in transgender patients. While buccal mucosa has become the graft material of choice in urethroplasty, patients who have undergone multiple reconstructive procedures require alternative sources of grafts.

I am deeply grateful to the world experts in reconstructive urology who took time away from their busy clinical practices to contribute these insightful articles.

Lee C. Zhao, MD, MS
Department of Urology
NYU Langone Medical Center
New York University School of Medicine
150 East 32nd Street, Second Floor
New York, NY 10016, USA

E-mail address:
Lee.zhao@nyumc.org

Urol Clin N Am 44 (2017) xv
http://dx.doi.org/10.1016/j.ucl.2016.10.001
0094-0143/17/© 2016 Published by Elsevier Inc.

urologic.theclinics.com

Definition of Successful Treatment and Optimal Follow-up after Urethral Reconstruction for Urethral Stricture Disease

Bradley A. Erickson, MD, MS*,
George M. Ghareeb, MD, MBA

KEYWORDS

- Urethroplasty • Urethral stricture • Stricture recurrence • Urethroplasty success
- Urethroplasty follow-up

KEY POINTS

- The traditional academic definition of a successful urethroplasty, lack of need for a secondary procedure, is outdated and should be amended to incorporate both objective (anatomic) and subjective (functional) outcomes measures.
- Anatomic success is assigned if a flexible cystoscope is able to traverse the reconstructed urethra without force during postoperative cystoscopy.
- Functional success is assigned if analysis of patient-reported outcome measures (PROMs) reveals improvement in voiding symptoms and urinary quality of life, without de novo sexual dysfunction or genitourinary pain.
- The optimal follow-up strategy must allow for determination of both anatomic and functional outcomes, protect patients' genitourinary health, and prevent patients from undergoing excessive invasive testing that leads to unnecessary cost, discomfort, anxiety, and risk.
- Objective uroflowmetry combined with PROMs and/or an obstructive voiding curve has high sensitivity and specificity for detecting recurrences and can be used as a surrogate for anatomic evaluation over time.

INTRODUCTION

Background

Male urethral stricture disease (USD) has an estimated prevalence of 0.6%.[1] The most typical way men present with USD is with obstructive voiding symptoms (eg, slow urinary flow).[2] However, up to 10% of patients will present without a history of bothersome symptoms and may only be diagnosed after a difficult urethral catheterization or during evaluation of recurrent urinary tract infections or urinary retention. USD can affect any part of the male urethra but most frequently affects the bulbar (43%) and penile (37%) segments.[3]

Treatment approaches for USD range from minimally invasive endoscopic techniques (eg, urethral dilation, direct visual internal urethrotomy) to open urethral reconstruction, which often uses local fasciocutaneous flaps and/or autologous tissue

Disclosure Statement: The above authors have nothing to disclose.
Department of Urology, University of Iowa Hospitals & Clinics, 200 Hawkins Drive, Iowa City, IA 52242, USA
* Corresponding author.
E-mail address: brad-erickson@uiowa.edu

Urol Clin N Am 44 (2017) 1–9
http://dx.doi.org/10.1016/j.ucl.2016.08.001
0094-0143/17/Published by Elsevier Inc.

grafts. Historical success rates for endoscopic management range from 0% to 50%,[4] with higher success rates being noted for shorter bulbar strictures that have not previously been managed surgically. Repeat endoscopic management is usually unsuccessful.[5] Open surgical techniques have significantly higher success rates, ranging from 50% to 98%,[3] with higher success rates generally being reported for shorter bulbar repairs that do not require flaps or grafts. Overall, success rates correlate well with the complexity of the repair.[6]

The most commonly performed treatments for USD continue to be endoscopic despite the lower reported success rates.[7] The apparent underuse of open urethral reconstruction in favor of endoscopic intervention is likely multifactorial, resulting from the relative simplicity of endoscopic techniques and the lack of familiarity and comfort with open techniques by many surgeons. Highlighting the educational deficits was a study by Bullock and Brandes,[7] which showed that, although 63% of urologists treated 6 to 20 urethral strictures in a given year, less than half of these urologists ever performed urethroplasty. In addition, side effects of urethroplasty, namely erectile dysfunction (ED) and urinary incontinence, are generally believed (falsely) to be more common than the literature supports, perhaps influencing both patient and provider enthusiasm for the procedures.[8]

Changing Practice Patterns for Urethral Stricture Disease

Attitudes about the treatment of USD seem to be changing, however, as demonstrated by a recently published article buy Liu and colleagues,[9] which showed a dramatic shift in the initial USD management over the past decade. The study revealed that, in 2004, urethroplasty was performed for USD only 2.3% of the time but, by 2012, the rate had increased to 7.6%. In addition, the years in practice seemed to be significantly associated with performance of urethroplasty, with newly certifying urologists being 3.7 times more likely to perform urethroplasty than their recertifying colleagues.[9] This change in attitudes is likely being spurred by a the rising number of Genitourinary Reconstructive Society fellowships in the United States,[10] more urethroplasties being performed in academic training centers, and the increase in academic interest in the field, particularly in outcomes of procedures that are performed to improve quality of life (ie, nononcologic surgeries).

Renewed academic interest in urethral reconstruction has forced the specialty to ask fundamental questions about the surgeries performed, the most basic of which is, "What constitutes a surgical success?" Traditionally, the academic definition of a successful urethroplasty has been defined as the lack of need for a secondary procedure. This definition is easily definable and, importantly, easy to quantitate using retrospective methodologies. However, the definition is also inherently subjective because it assumes that patient with recurrent symptoms will seek care at the center in which the urethroplasty was performed (ie, the patient did not go elsewhere for treatment); assumes equal utilization (both patient and provider) of secondary procedures for postoperative strictures; and, importantly, does not account for asymptomatic recurrences (ie, posturethroplasty decrease in urethral lumen size for which the patient does not have associated voiding symptoms), which have recently been shown to occur in up to 35% of recurrent strictures diagnosed by routine cystoscopy.[11]

Intimately associated with the question of how to define surgical success is the question "What is the best way to monitor the posturethroplasty patient?" With historical success rates being high and USD ultimately being a quality of life condition (ie, rarely does USD lead to mortality), excessive monitoring of the posturethroplasty patient is a legitimate concern because most urethroplasties will be ultimately be deemed successful. In addition, although academicians may be interested in topics such as postoperative urethral lumen size, most patients only care about their ability to empty their bladder in an appropriate and timely fashion. The ideal follow-up strategy must be able to account for both surgeon and patient concerns: maintaining the surgeon's ability to objectively define success (and failure) and protect patient's genitourinary health (ie, prevent bladder or renal dysfunction), all while preventing patients from undergoing unnecessary testing that leads to unnecessary cost, discomfort, anxiety, and risk.

Thus, the purpose of this article is 2-fold. This article reviews the literature for current definitions of surgical success and the current means by which the reconstructed urethra is monitored. It then proposes both a definition of success and a follow-up strategy that considers the concerns of both the patient and physician as previously listed.

DEFINING A SUCCESSFUL URETHROPLASTY

The basic goal of urethral reconstruction is to surgically construct a urethral lumen that is of large enough size (but not too large) to allow for the unimpeded flow of urine from the bladder through the urethra. Ultimately, the urethra provides little function other than acting as a conduit for socially acceptable expulsion of urine for both men and women. This is, perhaps, a major reason for the historical focus on the need or absence of need for secondary procedures when defining failure and success, respectively. However, as urethral reconstruction becomes a more acceptable early treatment of stricture disease and more physicians perform them nationwide, there is a collective realization beginning that patients expect more from an urethroplasty than just a larger lumen size.

Recent studies have shown that patient satisfaction after urethroplasty requires not only a decrease in the patient's postoperative urinary complaints (the traditional focus) but also an absence of pain and sexual side effects.[12] Thus, as surgeons become more interested in total patient experience after surgical procedures,[12] definitions of success need to be amended as well. Similar to a modern prostatectomy publication, in which a report of surgical margins and survival would be incomplete without a complementary report on postoperative incontinence and sexual dysfunction, the modern definition of urethroplasty success must also allow for both objective and subjective outcomes measures.

Absence of Secondary Procedures

A systematic review by Meeks and colleagues[3] revealed that 75% of the academic literature on urethral reconstruction published between 2000 and 2008 used the absence of a secondary procedure, regardless of urinary symptoms or the appearance of the reconstructed urethra, as the definition of surgical success. As previously noted, there are many logistical advantages to using such a definition; namely that this definition requires very little time or effort on either the patients' or the provider's part. However, this definition says very little about what is actually happening inside the urethral lumen (too big or too small?) or, for that matter, inside of patients' heads (ie, are they satisfied?). The definition also prevents surgeons from doing a true comparison between surgical techniques. For example, postvoid dribbling is a commonly reported postoperative complaint or complication after a few types of urethroplasties[13] but few surgeons would recommend a surgical procedure to correct it. Yet, should a patient with significant postvoid dribbling be considered a surgical success?

It is likely that, despite its limitations, this definition of success will remain popular both in practice and publications. However, this article attempts to show that, with risk stratification, urethroplasty specific objective follow-up, and patient-specific noninvasive follow-up strategies, this definition can potentially become more scientifically valid. Using a data-driven, standardized follow-up regimen will add more weight and significance in future publications to the cases of urethroplasty patients who have not undergone secondary procedures.

Objective Measurements

Cystoscopy and retrograde urethrogram (RUG) are objective means to monitor a reconstructed urethra and are often considered to be the gold standard follow-up methodologies. A flexible cystoscopy is easy to perform, relatively safe and is perhaps the most reliable way to compare the anatomy of a reconstructed urethra among patients and between centers. RUG has a few advantages compared with cystoscopy in that it can visualize the entire urethra simultaneously, may be able to more easily diagnose diverticula and fistulas, and is easier to compare to preoperative to postoperative objective findings. However, it is logistically difficult to perform in a standardized fashion and thus its interpretation can be considered subjective.

The Trauma and Urologic Reconstruction Network of Surgeons (TURNS; www.turns research.org), which is a network of 13 urologic reconstructive centers (and 14 surgeons) across the United States, uses a cystoscopy at 3 and 12 months to determine anatomic success, using the "inability to traverse the reconstructed urethra without force" as the definition of failure.[11] Using this protocol, the group found that 1-year success rates were significantly lower than had previously been reported (88.5% and 77.5% for excisional and substitutional repairs, respectively), likely due in large part to the nearly 35% of subjects with failure that were asymptomatic.[11] These are subjects with anatomic recurrences that would have been missed had the traditional definition of failure, secondary operations, been used, and thus reported success rates would have been much higher.

The cystoscopic protocol developed by the TURNS group was designed to be easily interpretable and reproducible across all centers. However, the findings perhaps created more questions than provided answers. For instance, what is the significance of the asymptomatic recurrences found in those subjects? Surgeons know that many classic obstructive symptoms will not generally develop until the urethral lumen is less than 16 F in size but does finding the recurrence early before symptoms develop offer long-term advantages to patients? Perhaps early detection (eg, for a distal graft recurrence) would prevent high intraurethral pressures within the graft but at what cost to the patient? Additionally, despite these subjects all consenting to the study protocol, compliance with 1-year cystoscopic follow-up was low, averaging only 54.4%, with many of subjects saying they did not follow-up because of a lack of symptoms, a lack of time, and in some cases, aversion to the impending cystoscopy.[11] Can a protocol in which nearly half of patients opt out really become a practical gold standard? Can surgical outcomes of a reconstructive procedure truly be compared without looking at the postoperative anatomy?

Noninvasive Objective Measurements

In the Meeks and colleagues[3] review, uroflowmetry (UF) was found to be performed in 56% of urethroplasty outcomes papers to screen for recurrence. UF is a noninvasive test that most commonly provides 3 metrics, maximum flow rate (Q_m), average flow rate (Q_a), and voided volume (VV), which can then be used to evaluate flow dynamics. The utility of the UF diminishes significantly (and is often disregarded) when the VV is less than 150 mL but, otherwise, VV is of little utility for screening purposes other than to help determine Q_m and Q_a.[14] The Q_m is the most widely cited measure to screen for recurrence, with many articles citing (arbitrarily) Q_m cut points ranging from 10 to 15 mL/s.[15] A postoperative patient with a flow below this threshold is generally then screened with cystoscopy or RUG for recurrence. However, although simple to understand and perform, UF has never been validated to be a very useful as a stand-alone tool for stricture recurrence screening.

The few studies that have specifically studied its utility have found that it works best when either combined with symptom analysis or when personalized to the specific patient. Erickson and colleagues[15] noted that using a Q_m of 10 mL/s in their postoperative subjects was only 54% sensitive at detecting recurrence. However, when UF was combined with symptoms and/or an obstructive voiding curve, the sensitivity increased to 99% (as did the negative predictive value) with an acceptable specificity of 98%.[15] This same group then analyzed subject-specific changes in Q_m and noted that when the Q_m increases by less than 10 mL/s postoperatively, these subjects are at high risk of recurrence.[14] In their retrospective cohort, had a ΔQ_m of less than 10 mL/s been used to screen for recurrence, it would have been 92% sensitive and 78% specific.[14] Importantly, these studies were retrospective in nature and were likely biased because subject follow-up

compliance was heavily influenced by the presence of symptoms. Another study by Heyns and Marais[16] noted that UF ($Q_m<15$) combined with the American Urologic Association Symptom Index (AUASI; total score>10) could help to predict strictures in untreated subjects, revealing a sensitivity of 93%, with a 68% specificity. However, this study did not specifically discuss its use in the postoperative patient.

A more recent study by Tam and Erickson and colleagues[17] evaluated the TURNS database and attempted to validate the routine use of UF specifically for diagnosing recurrence of stricture. The group found that a Q_m of less than 15 mL/s, a commonly cited cut-off in the literature when screening for urethroplasty, was only 41% sensitive for detecting cystoscopic recurrences (defined as the inability to traverse the urethroplasty site with a flexible cystoscopy).[17] However, the use of Q_m, and a novel parameter of $Q_m - Q_a$ (the value obtained when subtracting the Q_a value from Q_m), were significantly more useful in the postoperative period for men under 40 years of age.[17] Using receiver operating characteristic (ROC) curves, the group found the area under the curve (AUC) to be 0.932 and 0.922 for $Q_m - Q_a$ and Q_m, respectively in men younger than 40 years, as compared with 0.748 and 0.766 in men greater than 40.[17] The group hypothesized that this was likely because in younger men UF numbers are less influenced by the prostate and/or bladder dysfunction.[17] In addition, the group hypothesized that the $Q_m - Q_a$ parameter may be a useful numerical representation of the shape of the voiding curve, a somewhat subjective parameter that has been shown to be a useful indicator of obstruction compared with the Q_m value.

The measurement of the post-void residual (PVR), generally with the assistance of bladder ultrasound, has also been cited as a useful too when evaluating the reconstructed urethra, though generally as an adjunct to other noninvasive measurements. In the Meeks and colleagues[3] study, only 8% of articles cited PVR as a way to screen for recurrence after urethroplasty. However, because PVR depends on the hydration status of the patient, the timing of the last void relative to the test performance, the familiarity with the ultrasound machine by the tester, body habitus of the patient, and the variability in measurement algorithms by individual ultrasound machines, PVR is unlikely to ever become a useful stand-alone tool to monitor the reconstructed urethra. It may be useful, however, in identifying urethral stricture patients at risk for bladder failure (and potentially obstructive renal failure), though this is rare in younger population, most of whom can still empty their bladder even with USD.

Voiding Patient-Reported Outcomes Measures

For quality of life conditions such as USD, patient symptoms ultimately drive medical care. Urethral stricture patients will often seek care for obstructive voiding symptoms, such as urinary hesitancy and slow urinary flow. Thus, it seems reasonable to use validated patient-reported outcomes measures (PROMS) to evaluate urinary symptoms preoperatively and postoperatively, and to potentially use these PROMS to screen for recurrence because most patients would be expected to have new or persistent voiding symptoms.

One of the first studies to evaluate the use of a validated voiding questionnaire for screening purposes was conducted by Morey and colleagues,[18] showing that AUASI scores improved significantly after a successful urethroplasty. In this study, 9 out of 50 subjects had recurrence of their stricture and none of these subjects had significant improvements in their overall score postoperatively (as opposed to successful urethroplasties that decreased their score from 27 to 5), indicating that the AUASI may be useful for screening purposes.[18] In the Heyns and Marais[16] study mentioned previously, the addition of the AUASI score to the UF data improved the sensitivity to screen new USD.

Unfortunately, although it might be intuitive to think that all patients with recurrence of their stricture after urethroplasty would be symptomatic, a study of TURNS data by Erickson and colleagues[11] shows that many men with anatomic recurrence will be asymptomatic. In the study of 213 men, only 13 of 20 recurrences (65%) presented with urinary symptoms, implying that PROMS alone could miss recurrences in more than one-third of urethroplasty patients.[11] The potential limitations of PROM-only screening were recently validated in a study by Tam and colleagues.[19] Again, using TURNS data, the study revealed that after comparing the International Prostate Symptom Score (IPSS) to cystoscopy findings, the IPSS was only 50% sensitive in detecting anatomic recurrences when using a commonly used IPSS total score cutoff of 10.[19] Furthermore, on ROC analysis, single questions from the study (ie, urinary quality of life and weak stream) outperformed the total questionnaire (AUC 0.66 and 0.60 vs 0.56, respectively),[19] which emphasizes that, not only are these generic voiding questionnaires not helpful for USD patients, they fail to ask the specific questions that might be necessary to detect early recurrence (eg, "Has the strength of your urinary flow diminished since your catheter was initially removed?").

However, that approximately one-third of recurrences are asymptomatic begs the question, "what is the significance of the asymptomatic recurrence?" As previously stated, because USD is ultimately a quality of life condition, if the patient is without symptoms (and presumably in no danger of bladder and/or renal failure), why should surgeons care? The primary reason is that, without knowledge of the anatomic detail of the reconstructed urethra, different reconstructive options cannot be compared, such as between an excisional repair to a graft repair.

Nonvoiding Patient-Reported Outcomes Measures

Because open urethral reconstructive surgery involves surgery in the perineum and/or genitalia, patient concern for postoperative sexual dysfunction is understandably high. The reported rates of postoperative sexual dysfunction vary widely but a systematic review has shown that rates of permanent, de novo sexual dysfunction are likely around 1%.[20] However, transient ED has been reported to be as high as 40% at 3 months, with most studies showing improvement to baseline by 6 to 12 months.[21]

With such low rates of expected long-term ED, does it even need to be routinely assessed? The authors believe the need to fully compare different types of surgeries and different surgeons requires comparison of not just anatomic outcomes but factors that are important to the patient, including ED. A recent TURNS study that evaluated satisfaction after anterior urethroplasty depended on 3 factors independent of anatomic success: erectile function, pain, and voiding symptoms. Therefore, even if the surgeon created a widely patent urethra, if the patient had ED (even transient), new pain, or they did not perceive their urinary function to be improved, they were unhappy. Thus, these nonvoiding parameters should be a standard part of any complete urethroplasty follow-up to allow for assessment of the entire postoperative outcome.

Unfortunately, a standardized, validated questionnaire that assesses many of these symptoms does not exist specifically for anterior urethroplasty. The Jackson and colleagues[22] questionnaire assesses many voiding and quality of life measures. The questions, most of which were adopted from other questionnaires, were validated for the population but it was not developed with patient input. Newer questionnaires are currently in development that aim to take a more patient-centered approach to determining surgical outcomes.[23]

WHAT IS A SUCCESSFUL URETHROPLASTY?

Given how important, though often discordant, both the anatomic findings and patient-reported findings are in determining success after urethroplasty, the authors strongly believe that these parameters should be reported separately, and simultaneously, for all urethroplasty outcomes studies (**Table 1**). This modification in success rates reporting will make it easier to compare surgical outcomes between different surgeries, different surgeons, and different types of strictures.

Preoperative Evaluation

The suggested follow-up algorithm is shown in **Table 2**. To allow for personalization of the follow-up strategy, all patients should undergo PROM testing preoperatively and have a baseline UF study. Although there are no PROMs that were specifically designed for USD, the authors believe that a questionnaire, or set of questionnaires, that adequately assesses lower urinary tract symptoms (both voiding and storage, including postvoid dribbling), lower urinary tract pain, sexual function (including erectile and ejaculatory function), and quality of life are necessary.

Postoperative Evaluation

After performance of the urethroplasty that best suits the patient's stricture (and best follows the recently published American Urological Association urethroplasty guidelines)[24] and, after the operative catheter is removed (generally after a pericatheter RUG and/or voiding cystourethrogram confirms no contrast extravasation), patients should return to clinic for their initial postoperative evaluation between 3 and 6 months after surgery. The authors believe the timing of the initial postoperative evaluation is critical because most surgical healing has taken place by this time and any problems with initial graft or flap take will likely be evident.

Cystoscopy is the preferred method for objective follow-up at the initial clinic visit because it allows for direct inspection of the reconstructed urethral lumen. It also allows surgeons to provide a standardized way to compare their own operations over time and with other institutions. If a standard flexible cystoscope can traverse the urethral reconstruction without force, this constitutes an anatomic success. Before performance of the cystoscopy, a UF study should be obtained with a full bladder. Although UF alone is not adequate to diagnose stricture recurrence in the general population (see previous discussion), a UF at the time of cystoscopy can provide patient-specific UF parameters that can then be followed longitudinally. In essence, the initial postoperative UF study should serve as a patient's new baseline voiding parameters. A future significant decline (25%–30%) in the patient-specific Q_m or the $Q_m - Q_a$ should then prompt a repeat cystoscopic evaluation of the urethra, even in the absence of symptoms, to screen for anatomic recurrence.

Routine repeat cystoscopy at a year or later should be left to the surgeon discretion. The authors tend to perform routine yearly cystoscopy in higher risk patients (those with long grafts and/or flaps) and in patients with evidence of urethral narrowing (though not narrow enough to be considered recurrence) on their 3-month surveillance cystoscopy. However, routine cystoscopy at 1 year may be especially useful for physicians who do not perform many urethroplasties. Recent studies have revealed a significant learning curve for urethroplasty,[25] so visualizing the reconstructed urethra can provide valuable feedback for subsequent operations.

All patients should complete postoperative PROM questionnaires at each follow-up visit to allow for patient-specific symptom comparisons over time. Significant changes in PROM measures, including recent urinary tract infections, should prompt the urologist to consider objective evaluation of the urethra, especially if accompanied by a change in the patient-specific UF parameters.

Assigning Anatomic Success

An anatomic success should initially be assigned only after performance of a postoperative cystoscopy in which the flexible cystoscope is able to

Table 1
Proposed urethroplasty outcomes combining functional and anatomic outcomes

| | | Anatomic Evaluation Outcome | |
		Success	Failure
Functional Evaluation	Success	A	B
Outcome	Failure	C	D

A, percentage of patients with both functional and anatomic successes; B, percentage with functional success and anatomic failure (ie, asymptomatic recurrences); C, percentage with functional failure and anatomic success; D, percentage with both functional and anatomic failures (see **Fig. 1**).

Table 2
Urethral stricture disease treatment timeline and posturethroplasty follow-up protocol detailing assessment of functional and anatomic success

Phase of Care	Timing	Outcome Evaluation	
		Functional	**Anatomical**
Preoperative	Preoperative appointment	PROM Questionnaire[a]	• Baseline UF[b] • RUG and/or VCUG
Postoperative	3 wk		Pericatheter RUG and/or VCUG[c]
	3–6 mo (See **Fig. 1** for outcome determination algorithm)	PROM Questionnaire[d]	• UF before cystoscopy (new baseline)[e] • Cystoscopy (preferred) or RUG and/or VCUG
	12–15 mo	PROM Questionnaire	• UF • Need for cystoscopy (preferred) or RUG and/or VCUG per surgeon discretion[f]
	Annual follow-up thereafter	PROM Questionnaire	UF

Abbreviation: VCUG, voiding cystourethrogram.

[a] To evaluate for baseline voiding dysfunction (storage, elimination, postvoid dribbling), pain, and sexual functioning (erectile function, ejaculatory function).

[b] To assess voiding parameters of Q_m, Q_a, $Q_m - Q_a$, and evaluate voiding curve for obstructive pattern.

[c] To rule out contrast extravasation before catheter removal.

[d] To be compared with preoperative responses and assess for functional success.

[e] Serves as new baseline and can be followed over time as surrogate for anatomic evaluation if no anatomic failure on 3 to 6 month cystoscopy.

[f] Anatomic evaluation is recommended for high-risk patients (long strictures, flap, or graft), those with narrowing but not recurrence on 3–6 month cystoscopy, and lower volume surgeons.

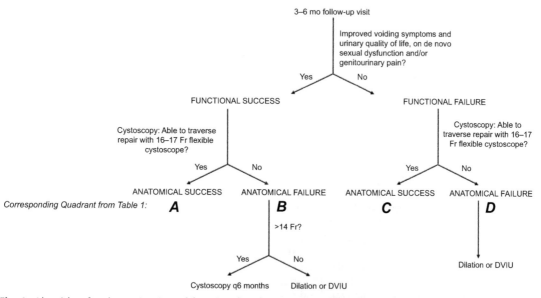

Fig. 1. Algorithm for determination of functional and anatomic success or failure. (*A*) Patients with both functional and anatomic successes corresponding to left-upper quadrant of outcomes reporting table (see **Table 1**). (*B*) Patients with functional success and anatomic failure (ie, asymptomatic recurrences) corresponding to right-upper quadrant. (*C*) Patients with functional failure and anatomic success corresponding to left-lower quadrant. (*D*) Patients with both functional and anatomic failures corresponding to right-lower quadrant. DVIU, direct vision internal urethrotomy.

traverse the reconstructed urethra without force (**Fig. 1**). Even in the setting of an asymptomatic patient, the inability to traverse the reconstruction with a standard (generally 16–17 F in size) cystoscope must be noted as an anatomic recurrence for the purposes of comparison. In these situations, the necessity of a secondary procedure is unclear but the authors suggest that any patient with increasing PVRs and bothersome urinary symptoms should have an intervention (endoscopic and/or revision urethroplasty).

After the initial anatomic evaluation with cystoscopy, the same-day UF studies can act as a surrogate to repeat cystoscopy for any patient with initial 3-month anatomic success. A decrease in the Q_m or $Q_m - Q_a$ (generally 20%–30%, though this has yet to be validated) should prompt an evaluation of the urethra with or without voiding symptoms.

Overall, the authors propose that anatomic success be used as a metric to compare the ability for various operations to create a durable lumen through which urine can effectively be expelled from the body. The authors also suggest that studies that report anatomic success in this manner should also report specific details about surgical technique (eg, suture type, suture technique) to further aid in study comparison and to improve the ability for surgeons to implement techniques in their own practice.

Assigning Functional Success

A functional success should be assigned after analysis of the postoperative PROMs. Functional success can occur in the setting of an anatomic failure and vice versa (see **Fig. 1**). The TURNS 1-year outcomes study revealed that up to 35% of patients without voiding symptoms can have anatomic (cystoscopic) failure[11] and many of these patients are satisfied with their repair and do not elect to have (or need) secondary operations.

The authors propose that assigning functional success should occur only after the following criteria are met: (1) bothersome voiding symptoms (directly attributable to the urethral stricture) have resolved or have not developed (eg, postvoid dribbling), (2) preoperative sexual function is preserved or improved, and (3) preoperative voiding and/or perioperative surgical pain has resolved. Unlike anatomic success rates, which might be expected to worsen with time, functional success rates will likely improve as has been shown by studies on both pain[26] and erectile function.[27]

PROM questionnaires should be completed by patients at each postoperative visit to allow for longitudinal comparison. Baseline PROM values should be obtained at the time of a normal cystoscopy so that any worsening of patient-specific voiding symptoms (especially obstructive symptoms, such as slow urinary flow and incomplete emptying) will increase the likelihood that interventional testing will reveal recurrence. This personalized approach to stricture monitoring will minimize the number of unnecessary invasive tests and represents a cost-effective approach to urethroplasty monitoring similar to strategies proposed by other groups.[28]

Overall, the authors propose that functional success should become a second, independently reported outcome measure by which surgical techniques can be adequately compared. Historical success rates have effectively concluded that all urethroplasties are created equal.[29] However, the authors strongly believe that utilization of this second outcome measure will reveal differences in the techniques that will help guide reconstructive urologists toward improved overall outcomes, especially in the factors that are important to patients.

SUMMARY

Urethral reconstruction has firmly established itself as the preferred method for the durable treatment of male USD. Although there are a multitude of techniques available for reconstruction that differ in their ability to treat strictures of varying lengths and locations, the ability to compare outcomes between the techniques has been hampered by the lack of a standardized definition of success and a standardized follow-up regimen. This article analyzes the available literature on the topics and proposes a 2-tiered definition of success that considers both anatomic and functional factors, and offers a personalized follow-up strategy that will improve the ability to report success, detect recurrence, and minimize unnecessary invasive testing.

REFERENCES

1. Alwaal A, Blaschko SD, McAninch JW, et al. Epidemiology of urethral strictures. Transl Androl Urol 2014;3(2):209–13.
2. Mundy AR, Andrich DE. Urethral strictures. BJU Int 2011;107(1):6–26.
3. Meeks JJ, Erickson BA, Granieri MA, et al. Stricture recurrence after urethroplasty: a systematic review. J Urol 2009;182(4):1266–70.
4. Pansadoro V, Emiliozzi P. Internal urethrotomy in the management of anterior urethral strictures: long-term followup. J Urol 1996;156(1):73–5.
5. Heyns CF, Steenkamp JW, De Kock ML, et al. Treatment of male urethral strictures: is repeated dilation

or internal urethrotomy useful? J Urol 1998;160(2): 356–8.

6. Alwaal A, Sanford TH, Harris CR, et al. Urethral Stricture Score is Associated with Anterior Urethroplasty Complexity and Outcome. J Urol 2016; 195(6):1817–21.

7. Bullock TL, Brandes SB. Adult anterior urethral strictures: a national practice patterns survey of board certified urologists in the United States. J Urol 2007;177(2):685–90.

8. Patel DP, Elliott SP, Voelzke BB, et al. Patient-reported sexual function after staged penile urethroplasty. Urology 2015;86(2):395–400.

9. Liu JS, Hofer MD, Oberlin DT, et al. Practice Patterns in the Treatment of Urethral Stricture Among American Urologists: A Paradigm Change? Urology 2015;86(4):830–4.

10. Erickson BA, Voelzke BB, Myers JB, et al. Practice patterns of recently fellowship-trained reconstructive urologists. Urology 2012;80(4):934–7.

11. Erickson BA, Elliott SP, Voelzke BB, et al. Multi-institutional 1-year bulbar urethroplasty outcomes using a standardized prospective cystoscopic follow-up protocol. Urology 2014;84(1):213–6.

12. Bertrand LA, Voelzke BB, Elliott SP, et al. Measuring and Predicting Patient Dissatisfaction after Anterior Urethroplasty Using Patient Reported Outcomes Measures. J Urol 2016;196(2):453–61.

13. Barbagli G, Voelzke BB, Elliott SP, et al. Muscle- and nerve-sparing bulbar urethroplasty: a new technique. Eur Urol 2008;54(2):335–43.

14. Erickson BA, Breyer BN, McAninch JW. Changes in uroflowmetry maximum flow rates after urethral reconstructive surgery as a means to predict for stricture recurrence. J Urol 2011;186(5):1934–7.

15. Erickson BA, Breyer BN, McAninch JW. The use of uroflowmetry to diagnose recurrent stricture after urethral reconstructive surgery. J Urol 2010;184(4): 1386–90.

16. Heyns CF, Marais DC. Prospective evaluation of the American Urological Association symptom index and peak urinary flow rate for the followup of men with known urethral stricture disease. J Urol 2002; 168(5):2051–4.

17. Tam CA, Voelzke BB, Elliott SP, et al. Critical Analysis of the Use of Uroflowmetry for Urethral Stricture Disease Surveillance. Urology 2016;91:197–202.

18. Morey AF, McAninch JW, Duckett CP, et al. American Urological Association symptom index in the assessment of urethroplasty outcomes. J Urol 1998;159(4):1192–4.

19. Tam CA, Elliott SP, Voelzke BB, et al. The International Prostate Symptom Score (IPSS) Is an Inadequate Tool to Screen for Urethral Stricture Recurrence After Anterior Urethroplasty. Urology 2016;95:197–201.

20. Blaschko SD, Sanford MT, Cinman NM, et al. De novo erectile dysfunction after anterior urethroplasty: a systematic review and meta-analysis. BJU Int 2013;112(5):655–63.

21. Erickson BA, Wysock JS, McVary KT, et al. Erectile function, sexual drive, and ejaculatory function after reconstructive surgery for anterior urethral stricture disease. BJU Int 2007;99(3):607–11.

22. Jackson MJ, Chaudhury I, Mangera A, et al. A prospective patient-centred evaluation of urethroplasty for anterior urethral stricture using a validated patient-reported outcome measure. Eur Urol 2013; 64(5):777–82.

23. Voelzke BB, Edwards TC, Patrick DL, et al. PD16–03 patient and clinician prioritization of outcomes among men with anterior urethral stricture disease. J Urol 2016;195(4):e395.

24. Male Urethral Stricture: AUA Guideline, in Male Urethral Stricture: AUA Guideline, A.U. Association, editor. 2016. Available at: https://www.auanet.org/common/pdf/education/clinical-guidance/Male-Urethral-Stricture.pdf.

25. Faris SF, Myers JB, Voelzke BB, et al. Assessment of the Male Urethral Reconstruction Learning Curve. Urology 2016;89:137–43.

26. Bertrand LA, Warren GJ, Voelzke BB, et al. Lower urinary tract pain and anterior urethral stricture disease: prevalence and effects of urethral reconstruction. J Urol 2015;193(1):184–9.

27. Erickson BA, Granieri MA, Meeks JJ, et al. Prospective analysis of ejaculatory function after anterior urethral reconstruction. J Urol 2010;184(1): 238–42.

28. Belsante MJ, Zhao LC, Hudak SJ, et al. Cost-effectiveness of risk stratified followup after urethral reconstruction: a decision analysis. J Urol 2013; 190(4):1292–7.

29. Chen ML, Odom BD, Santucci RA. Substitution urethroplasty is as successful as anastomotic urethroplasty for short bulbar strictures. Can J Urol 2014; 21(6):7565–9.

Cost-effective Strategies for the Management and Treatment of Urethral Stricture Disease

CrossMark

E. Charles Osterberg, MD[a], Gregory Murphy, MD[a],
Catherine R. Harris, MD[a,b], Benjamin N. Breyer, MD, MAS[a,*]

KEYWORDS

- Urethroplasty • Cost-effectiveness • Utilization

KEY POINTS

- Urethroplasty is a cost-effective strategy for operative management of urethral stricture disease.
- An accurate estimation of stricture recurrence will guide urologists toward the appropriate intervention.
- Symptom-based surveillance of postoperative urethral stricture disease will reduce unnecessary diagnostic procedures and cost.

INTRODUCTION

Urethral stricture disease (USD) is a narrowing of the urethra from scar tissue, attributed to traumatic urethral injury, infections of the genitourinary tract, pelvic radiation, inflammatory skin conditions, and/or prior lower urinary tract instrumentation.[1] USD causes both obstructive and irritative voiding symptoms and can result in bladder and renal impairment.[1] The prevalence of USD among men from industrialized countries is estimated to be 0.9%.[1] In the United States between 2007 and 2012, an estimated 1.2 million patients sought medical care for USD.[2]

Treatment options for USD include endoscopic and/or open surgical techniques. The mainstay for endoscopic managements include urethral dilation or direct vision internal urethrotomy (DVIU). Open reconstructive surgical techniques include urethroplasty, which may be performed in conjunction with a graft or flap.[1] The management of USD

has shifted from periodic dilation to DVIU and now urethroplasty, as the definitive procedure of choice for recurrent USD.[3,4] Although DVIU may be used for short, bulbar strictures,[5] its long-term efficacy has been called into question.[6] Urethroplasty is considered to be the gold standard for USD and has high success rates.[7] Despite the convincing evidence for urethroplasty, a recent Cochrane review concluded that there are insufficient data to determine which intervention is best for USD in terms of balancing efficacy, adverse effects, and costs.[8]

To date, many urologists report repeating a DVIU or dilation procedure despite the high rate of recurrence.[9] Repeated endoscopic interventions for recurrent USD are futile and have been proven to be cost-ineffective.[3,4,10] Estimates of procedural costs for USD are limited.[11] With the passage of the Affordable Care Act and paradigm shift toward cost-effective medicine, urologists are urged to perform efficacious procedures at lower

Conflict of Interests: None.
[a] Department of Urology, University of California, San Francisco, 400 Parnassus Ave, San Francisco, CA 94143, USA; [b] Department of Urology, Stanford University, 300, Palo Alto, CA 94304, USA
* Corresponding author. 1001 Potrero Avenue, Suite 3A, San Francisco, CA 94110.
E-mail address: Benjamin.breyer@ucsf.edu

costs.[12] There is an increased attention toward high-value, low-cost health care in the United States as the projected cost of current practices may be unsustainable.[13] Policy makers, government officials, and insurance companies have scrutinized procedural costs and surgical outcomes to maximize quality care at lower costs.[14] Such scrutiny has led to the development of quality reporting clearinghouses like the American Urologic Association Quality Registry and the National Surgical Quality Improvement Program.[14,15]

Within the last 10 years, several studies have been published on cost-effective management strategies for USD as part of a growing focus on high-quality, low-cost health care. Here the authors present a review of current literature on minimizing cost for patients with USD. In particular, the authors focus on the costs of managing USD with DVIU versus urethroplasty, inpatient hospital costs following urethroplasty, and the costs of USD surveillance strategies.

COST OF INTERNAL URETHROTOMY/ DILATION VERSUS URETHROPLASTY

In 1974, optical DVIU was first reported and quickly gained acceptance because of its simplicity, reliability, safety, and short convalescence.[9] Today, urologists use either a cold-knife or a laser source to perform cuts within the urethra at the level of the stricture. Although initial reports suggested short-term success to be around 80%,[16] it is well known that the success of DVIU is much lower with longer follow-up and well-designed prospective studies.[5,17] In patients with at least 60 months of follow-up, DVIU was found to be successful in only 32% of men.[5] Urethral dilation has a similar success, as several studies have shown dilation to be equal in efficacy to DVIU.[17,18] Nevertheless, DVIU remains the most common procedure performed for USD in the United States.[19] In a nationwide survey, 31% of urologists reported repeating a second DVIU after the first failed DVIU.[9] However, DVIU has been proven to be cost-ineffective in several well-reported studies.

In 2004, Greenwell and colleagues[3] developed an algorithm for the management of USD based on cost-effectiveness. The investigators used the UK's medical insurance reimbursement rates and applied them to 126 men treated for USD over an 8-year period. Men with preexisting USD that previously required intervention were excluded from the study. The investigators followed patients for a mean of 25 months (range 1–132 months). Of the 126 men with a new diagnosis of USD, 60 (47.6%) required more than 1 endoscopic treatment (mean 3.13 treatments). In total, 194 additional procedures were performed for recurrent USD, of which 7 were urethroplasties. The investigators calculated the total costs of care for USD over their follow-up period by multiplying the number of procedures by the costs of endoscopic treatments, the costs associated with clean intermittent catheterization, and ultimately the costs associated with urethroplasty. They concluded that the total cost per patient with USD was $9170; however, this cost could be lowered if urethral dilation or DVIU was performed as a first-line treatment and then subsequent urethroplasty was performed for recurrent USD. In doing so, the cost per patient would be reduced to $8799.[3] Despite a theoretic savings of $371 if urethroplasty was performed after endoscopic failure, the article has several limitations. The investigators presumed a second-stage urethroplasty would require only 2 postoperative visits; they assumed the hospital length of stay for all patients to be standard (24-hour hospital stay for DVIU or dilation, 3 days for simple urethroplasty, and 5 days for complex urethroplasty); the investigators assumed a ratio of first- to second-stage urethroplasties to be 1.9:1.0; and lastly they assumed a 10.5% stricture recurrence rate, both figures derived from their historical data. They also included data from both bulbar and penile urethral strictures, which are not comparable groups. Each of these factors could dramatically alter the costs of USD.

In 2005, Rourke and Jordan[4] constructed a decision model using decisional analysis (DA). Briefly, DA is a statistical method whereby a systematic framework for decision-making is applied between 2 competing options. One outcome of a DA is a cost-effectiveness ratio that attempts to maximize the outcome for a given budget.[10] In this study, the investigators used published data on the costs of bleeding, urinary tract infection, and stricture recurrence following DVIU and compared this with published data on the costs of a wound complication, complications from high lithotomy positioning, and stricture recurrence. The primary aim was to determine the least costly approach for a hypothetical male patient seeking treatment of a 2-cm bulbar urethral stricture.[4] Cost estimates for the postoperative complications, surgeon's fees, hospital fees, operative costs, and costs of follow-up procedures were based on Medicare reimbursement and data from the investigators' home institutions. Total costs for DVIU were calculated to be $17,748 versus $16,444 for anastomotic urethroplasty yielding a cost savings of $1304 per patient. Only when a theoretic success of DVIU approached

60% did the procedure become cost-effective.[4] Similarly, as long as the theoretic success of urethroplasty remained more than 71%, then it was more cost-effective; most large series report urethroplasty success to be much higher.[20] Despite a clear monetary difference between procedures, it is unclear that this would generalize to a prospective series of patients. Furthermore, the investigators point that that they used estimates of costs based on their own institution's data and surgeries were performed by high-volume surgeons. The investigators also point that their study failed to analyze outcomes and, thus, the cost-effectiveness of different interventions cannot be determined unless the effectiveness of the alternatives is assumed to be similar. Nevertheless, the up-front cost of urethroplasty, although costlier, has a higher success rate.

In **Table 1**, the authors summarize data based on Greenwell and colleagues[3] and Rourke and Jordan.[4] For simplicity sake, the authors assume that urethroplasty is highly successful (eg, ~100%). The authors demonstrate that the combined cost of a failed DVIU procedure followed by a urethroplasty is higher than the up-front cost of urethroplasty alone.

Using a similar DA, Wright and colleagues[10] published data in 2006 comparing the costs of different management strategies for a 1- to 2-cm bulbar stricture. The authors constructed a decision tree whereby the number of planned DVIUs was hypothesized before planned urethroplasty. Fees associated with procedural costs derived from Medicare data, office visits, and lost wages from convalescence were collected. The authors found that for a 1- to 2-cm bulbar stricture, with published success rate of 50% for the first DVIU, 20% for the second DVIU, and 95% for anastomotic urethroplasty, a strategy of one DVIU preceding urethroplasty was least costly ($8575) compared with 2 DVIUs followed by urethroplasty ($9285) or up-front urethroplasty ($10,222). When

first-time DVIU success was estimated to be less than 35%, up-front urethroplasty was most cost-effective.[10] This finding differs from the study by Rourke and Jordan[4] because of the differing rates of success and cost estimates.

Taking the 3 aforementioned studies together, as the success of a DVIU decreases, the most cost-effective option for USD is urethroplasty. In **Fig. 1**, the authors demonstrated that the theoretic cost per patient is inversely proportional to the success rate of the procedure. As DVIU becomes more successful, it is cheaper on a population level or per patient and the same is true for urethroplasty. In either case, the failures are costly. Perhaps the most challenging aspect of determining cost-effectiveness of urethroplasty over DVIU is an accurate prediction of success and recurrence rates. Given the heterogeneity of data, urologists who treat USD must choose the appropriate and cost-effective procedure after weighing a patients' presenting symptoms, their proposed outcomes, predicted success, existing comorbidities, predicted postoperative convalesce, and patient preferences (**Fig. 2**). Here, expert clinical judgment is essential to guide patients to the most appropriate surgery. For example, a straddle injury-induced stricture has a notoriously high restricture rate following DVIU due to dense focal spongiofibrosis and is unlikely to respond to DVIU.[21] In this instance, clinical acumen and understanding of USD is key to providing cost-effective, efficacious patient care.

UNDERUTILIZATION OF URETHROPLASTY

Despite studies demonstrating improved efficacy and cost-effectiveness of urethroplasty over DVIU, there remains high regional variation using urethroplasty within the United States. Using claims from MarketScan data, Figler and colleagues[19] found that endoscopic management of USD was far more common than urethroplasty.

Table 1
Success and cost of urethroplasty versus direct vision internal urethrotomy

First Treatment	Cost	Success Rate (%)	Second Treatment	Cost	Success Rate (%)	Cost Per Patient
DVIU	$3375.00	28	Urethoplasty	$7522.5	~100	$8791.20
Urethoplasty	$7722.50	96	2-Stage urethroplasty	$15,555.00	~100	$8144.70
DVIU	$3375.00	28	Lifelong intermittent catheterization	$17.00/mo	0	$8144.70

Data from Greenwell TJ, Castle C, Andrich DE, et al. Repeat urethrotomy and dilation for the treatment of urethral stricture are neither clinically effective nor cost-effective. J Urol 2004;172(1):275–7; and Rourke KF, Jordan GH. Primary urethral reconstruction: the cost minimized approach to the bulbous urethral stricture. J Urol 2005;173(4):1206–10.

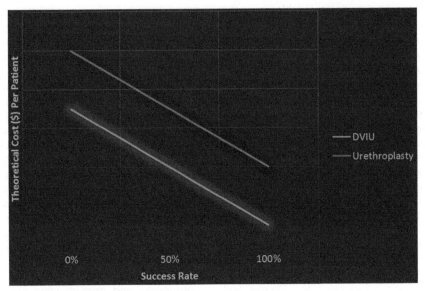

Fig. 1. Cost-effectiveness of DVIU versus urethroplasty.

Those patients who underwent urethroplasty were younger, more likely to travel to a metropolitan area for treatment, and a reconstructive urologist was more likely to be involved in their treatment. Among the Veterans Affairs' hospital system, a similar phenomenon is seen whereby only 5% of men underwent a urethroplasty, and most underwent a DVIU or dilation.[22] Among the elderly, Anger and colleagues[23] demonstrate that Medicare beneficiaries are also more likely to undergo DVIU or dilation over a urethroplasty despite increasing trends in USD. Review of the American Board of Urology's surgical case logs demonstrated that urologists performed 17 DVIU or dilations per every 1 urethroplasty.[24] These trends are attributable to several factors, including an unfamiliarity of published outcomes of urethroplasty[9] and a lack of qualified reconstructive urologists in certain regions of the United States, yet 74% of urologists think that urethroplasty should be offered after repeat endoscopic treatment failure.[19]

INPATIENT HOSPITAL COSTS ASSOCIATED WITH URETHROPLASTY

Although most endoscopic management of USD is performed in an outpatient setting, most urethroplasties performed in the United States are done with either a short stay or inpatient hospital admission.[25] Associated costs with hospital admission may challenge up-front urethroplasty over an initial DVIU attempt. Characterizing hospital costs associated with urethroplasty may better identify the major drivers of hospital costs associated with USD.

Blaschko and colleagues[2] used the National Inpatient Sample data to determine national trends of urethroplasties and costs associated with inpatient hospitalization. The investigators reported an overall complication rate of 6.6%, which increased with age and comorbidities but not type of urethroplasty performed. As the number of complications increased, the mean length of hospital stay and total charges rendered for the hospital stay increased. The mean total hospital charges were

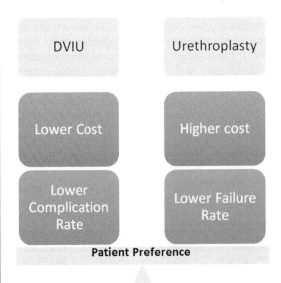

Fig. 2. Balancing efficacy and cost-effectiveness for DVIU versus urethroplasty.

3-fold higher for patients with 3 or more postoperative complications (from $24,853 to $77,059).[2] Interpretation of hospital costs associated with urethroplasty is limited because the investigators did not control for length of stay or complexity of urethroplasty.

To gain a more granular assessment of inpatient costs associated with urethroplasty, Harris and colleagues[25] used the same data set but captured hospital charges relating to USD. Over the investigators' study period, a total of 2298 urethroplasties were performed with a median hospital cost of $7321. With extreme costs defined as the top 20th percentile of expenditure, the investigators found that patients with multiple comorbid diseases were associated with increased costs (odds ratio [OR] 1.56, 95% confidence interval [CI] 1.19–2.04, P = .02).[25] Inpatient complications increased the odds of extreme costs (OR 3.2 95% CI 2.14–4.75, P <.001), as did graft urethroplasties (OR 1.78, 95% CI 1.2–2.64, P = .005). Interestingly, the investigators did not find any differences in extreme costs based on patient age, race, hospital region, bed size, teaching status, payer type, and volume of urethroplasty cases.[25] Although the study was limited to inpatient/short-stay hospital-associated costs, the major drivers of costs associated with urethroplasty stem from postoperative complications and to a lesser degree from preoperative patient comorbidities and surgical complexity. Currently, the total costs of outpatient urethroplasty have not been reported in the literature. Future studies should compare an in-depth analysis of outpatient urethroplasty stratified by stricture location/complexity.

COSTS OF FOLLOW-UP AFTER URETHROPLASTY

The cost-effectiveness of urethroplasty for recurrent USD may be sustained by the prolonged stricture-free rates. This highly efficacious procedure will allow for decreased postoperative follow-up visits. With recurrence rates after DVIU as high as 80%, patients will often require repeat office evaluation, diagnostic retrograde urethrograms, and cystoscopies.[5] For urethroplasty, despite a lower recurrence, patients will also undergo repeat office evaluation with diagnostic evaluation. Currently, there remains no standard surveillance approach for USD following urethroplasty. A wide range of both noninvasive (uroflowmetry, questionnaires, postvoid residual ultrasound, and so forth) and invasive (retrograde urethrogram, voiding cystourethrogram, urethral calibration, and cystoscopy) options is available for stricture surveillance.[26] In 2015, Zaid and

colleagues[26] surveyed current literature to delineate commonly used surveillance strategies and compared the costs of varying diagnostic evaluations used by urologists. The investigators reported that the median cost for the first year of USD surveillance following anterior urethroplasty was $660, and over 5 years this extrapolated to $1069. Following a posterior urethroplasty, the median cost of surveillance at 1 and 5 years was $800 and $1286, respectively. Most surveillance costs occurred in the first postoperative year.[26] This study demonstrates there is significant variability in the frequency and intensity of postoperative USD surveillance. Currently, there is no standard of surveillance that balances cost-conscious care with early diagnosis of recurrence. Furthermore, it is not known whether early diagnosis of USD recurrence following urethroplasty has been shown to improve clinical outcomes.

To demonstrate a cost-effective, risk-stratified approach to patient follow-up following urethroplasty, Belsante and colleagues[27] performed a DA demonstrating a reduction in unnecessary follow-up visits, invasive testing, and radiation exposures. In 2013, the investigators compared a hypothetical simplified, symptom-based follow-up protocol with a standard regimen of close follow-up following anastomotic urethroplasty. The two arms of the study included a low-risk, anastomotic urethroplasty group in which theoretic patients only followed up as needed and a standard-risk group, which included any flap/graft urethroplasty and/or a history of radiation, lichen sclerosus, or hypospadias. This hypothetical standard-risk group underwent a regimented follow-up protocol every 3 months for 1 year and then yearly after with a uroflowmetry and retrograde urethrogram. Using a simplified, symptom-based follow-up scheme of men who underwent anastomotic urethroplasty, Belsante and colleagues[27] found that it was 85% lower in cost versus a regimented follow-up practice ($430 vs $2827) for standard patients. Using sensitivity analysis, the investigators concluded that when the success rate of anastomotic urethroplasty was greater than 10%, a symptom-based follow-up was most cost-effective. The rationale for the authors' conclusion is that recurrent USD will manifest with lower urinary tract symptoms, and unnecessary diagnostic testing is of little benefit to patients.[27] Therefore, stratifying USD by risk of recurrence will greatly decrease the burden of follow-up and cost.

SUMMARY

When considering the most cost-effective option for men with USD, a surgeon must rely on his or her estimates of recurrence, complication rates, and convalescence. Current data suggest that urethroplasty is a more cost-effective procedure for USD, especially in patients who have failed DVIU. Costs for inpatient urethroplasty are mainly driven by postoperative complications and patient comorbidities. Standard surveillance regimens for USD recurrence are lacking; however, a simplified, symptom-based approach is more cost-conscious. The authors present current data that balances the accessibility and inexpensiveness of a DVIU with the long-term efficacy at a higher surgical cost for urethroplasty. In times of fiscal constraint and managed health care, it is imperative to evaluate surgical efficacy in terms of cost-saving strategies. Future studies should examine the cost-effectiveness of up-front urethroplasty and efficacy as compared with endoscopic management followed by urethroplasty. Well-designed, adequately powered, multicenter trials are also needed to prospectively evaluate if urethroplasty is more cost-effective over DVIU/dilation. As urologists, our duty is to improve our patients' quality of life by maximizing patient outcomes and experience in a cost-conscious manner.

REFERENCES

1. Tritschler S, Roosen A, Fullhase C, et al. Urethral stricture: etiology, investigation and treatments. Dtsch Arztebl Int 2013;110(13):220–6.

2. Blaschko SD, Harris CR, Zaid UB, et al. Trends, utilization, and immediate perioperative complications of urethroplasty in the United States: data from the national inpatient sample 2000-2010. Urology 2015;85(5):1190–4.

3. Greenwell TJ, Castle C, Andrich DE, et al. Repeat urethrotomy and dilation for the treatment of urethral stricture are neither clinically effective nor cost-effective. J Urol 2004;172(1):275–7.

4. Rourke KF, Jordan GH. Primary urethral reconstruction: the cost minimized approach to the bulbous urethral stricture. J Urol 2005;173(4):1206–10.

5. Pansadoro V, Emiliozzi P. Internal urethrotomy in the management of anterior urethral strictures: long-term follow-up. J Urol 1996;156(1):73–5.

6. Heyns CF, Steenkamp JW, De Kock ML, et al. Treatment of male urethral strictures: is repeated dilation or internal urethrotomy useful? J Urol 1998;160(2):356–8.

7. Mundy AR, Andrich DE. Urethral strictures. BJU Int 2011;107(1):6–26.

8. Wong SS, Narahari R, O'Riordan A, et al. Simple urethral dilatation, endoscopic urethrotomy, and urethroplasty for urethral stricture disease in adult men. Cochrane Database Syst Rev 2010;(4): CD006934.

9. Bullock TL, Brandes SB. Adult anterior urethral strictures: a national practice patterns survey of board certified urologists in the United States. J Urol 2007;177(2):685–90.

10. Wright JL, Wessells H, Nathens AB, et al. What is the most cost-effective treatment for 1 to 2-cm bulbar urethral strictures: societal approach using decision analysis. Urology 2006;67(5):889–93.

11. Santucci RA, Joyce GF, Wise M. Male urethral stricture disease. J Urol 2007;177(5):1667–74.

12. Erickson BA. What is the role of cost-effectiveness analysis in clinical practice? J Urol 2013;190(4): 1163–4.

13. Antos J, Bertko J, Chernew M, et al. Bending the curve: effective steps to address long-term healthcare spending growth. Am J Manag Care 2009; 15(10):676–80.

14. Ingraham AM, Richards KE, Hall BL, et al. Quality improvement in surgery: the American College of Surgeons National Surgical Quality Improvement Program approach. Adv Surg 2010;44:251–67.

15. Association AU. AUA Quality (AQUA) Registry. 2016. Available at: https://www.auanet.org/resources/aqua.cfm.

16. Smith PJ, Dunn M, Dounis A. The early results of treatment of stricture of the male urethra using the Sachse optical urethrotome. Br J Urol 1979;51(3):224–8.

17. Santucci R, Eisenberg L. Urethrotomy has a much lower success rate than previously reported. J Urol 2010;183(5):1859–62.

18. Steenkamp JW, Heyns CF, de Kock ML. Internal urethrotomy versus dilation as treatment for male urethral strictures: a prospective, randomized comparison. J Urol 1997;157(1):98–101.

19. Figler BD, Gore JL, Holt SK, et al. High regional variation in urethroplasty in the United States. J Urol 2015;193(1):179–83.

20. Hampson LA, McAninch JW, Breyer BN. Male urethral strictures and their management. Nat Rev Urol 2014;11(1):43–50.

21. Wessells H. Cost-effective approach to short bulbar urethral strictures supports single internal urethrotomy before urethroplasty. J Urol 2009;181(3):954–5.

22. Anger JT, Scott VC, Sevilla C, et al. Patterns of management of urethral stricture disease in the Veterans Affairs system. Urology 2011;78(2):454–8.

23. Anger JT, Buckley JC, Santucci RA, et al. Urologic diseases in America P. trends in stricture management among male Medicare beneficiaries: underuse of urethroplasty? Urology 2011;77(2):481–5.

24. Burks FN, Salmon SA, Smith AC, et al. Urethroplasty: a geographic disparity in care. J Urol 2012;187(6): 2124–7.

25. Harris CR, Osterberg EC, Sanford T, et al. National variation in urethroplasty cost and predictors of

extreme cost: a cost analysis with policy implications. Urology 2016;94:246–54.

26. Zaid UB, Hawkins M, Wilson L, et al. The cost of surveillance after urethroplasty. Urology 2015;85(5):1195–9.

27. Belsante MJ, Zhao LC, Hudak SJ, et al. Cost-effectiveness of risk stratified follow-up after urethral reconstruction: a decision analysis. J Urol 2013; 190(4):1292–7.

Endoscopic Treatment of Urethral Stenosis

Brittney H. Cotta, MD, Jill C. Buckley, MD*

KEYWORDS

- Urethral stenosis • Endoscopic treatment • Urethral stricture disease • Urethral reconstruction

KEY POINTS

- Urethral stricture disease continues to be a common problem for patients and urologists alike.
- Endoscopic treatment offers a simple, potentially effective treatment of primary, short, urethral strictures.
- For patients who recur after endoscopic management, urethral or bladder neck reconstruction should be offered with an experienced urologic reconstructionist familiar with the complexity of the situation and subtleties of the surgery.
- With the advent of adjunctive antifibrotic agents the durability of endoscopic repair seems to improve, but their use requires continued research and longer follow-up to determine their efficacy.

INTRODUCTION

Urethral stricture disease is a common and challenging problem for general urologists and reconstructive urologists alike. Although strictures commonly present with similar symptoms of difficulty voiding, split urine stream, postvoid dribbling, or even urinary retention, urinary strictures may form in discrete areas along the urethra. As the cause and treatment varies between these subtypes, strictures can be best characterized as anterior urethral strictures, posterior urethral strictures, or bladder neck contractures.

In most instances, urethral strictures or bladder neck contractures (BNCs) are initially treated with an in-office dilation. However, this procedure is uncomfortable for patients, can be challenging for the urologist to perform, and generally is associated with high recurrence rates that require repeat intervention. When dilation fails, the next step is often a repeat urethral dilation (UD) or an internal urethrotomy (IU). IU is the type of procedure in which the stricture is opened by cold-knife incision or thermal energy incision performed transurethrally. The intent is to release/open the scar contracture through incision with the goal that generative healing occurs at a more rapid rate than scar formation.

Endoscopic treatment of stricture disease offers a minimally invasive approach with advantages over open surgery, such as its ability to be done as an outpatient or in the clinic, associated lower cost, and relative simplicity compared with urethroplasty. Despite these advantages, urethroplasty remains the most definitive treatment of stricture disease. Even in stricture types whereby endoscopic management has been shown to be most effective (short bulbar urethral strictures), stricture-free rates after urethroplasty are reported as high as 90% to 95%[1,2] versus 50% to 70%[3] for endoscopic treatment. In certain locations, such as distal or pendulous urethral strictures, the stricture-free rates of dilation or urethral incision are much lower, 30% or less, and should be viewed primarily as a palliative maneuver that will likely require life-long intervention. Endoscopic management has evolved from the single 12-o'clock IU originally described to numerous

Disclosure Statement: The authors have nothing to disclose.
Department of Urology, UC San Diego Health System, 200 West Arbor Drive, San Diego, CA 92103-8897, USA
* Corresponding author. Department of Urology, UC San Diego Health System, 200 West Arbor Drive, #8897, San Diego, CA 92103-8897.
E-mail address: jcbuckley@ucsd.edu

Urol Clin N Am 44 (2017) 19–25
http://dx.doi.org/10.1016/j.ucl.2016.08.008

variations in technique to create the most effective and durable endoscopic repair.

ANTERIOR URETHRAL STRICTURES

The anterior urethra is composed of the meatus to the proximal bulbar urethra. Anterior urethral strictures develop through a process called spongiofibrosis, wherein the urethral epithelial cells are damaged either by external or internal trauma, exposing the underlying corpus spongiosum. This exposure results in a dense collagen scar formed by fibroblasts and a narrowing due to external urethral pressure as the urethra attempts to repair itself. The resultant scar is further irritated by the passage of urine, causing even more spongiofibrosis.[4] The causes include idiopathic, iatrogenic, inflammatory, and traumatic,[5] which often occur in predictable locations.

Direct Vision Internal Urethrotomy

After dilation, the most commonly performed treatment of anterior urethral strictures is direct vision internal IU (DVIU). Sachse[6] first introduced DVIU of anterior urethral stenosis in 1974. Because of its minimally invasive approach and the familiarity of endoscopic procedures in urology, it has quickly become a go-to treatment of stricture disease such that in a survey of American Urologic Association members, 85.6% reported using DVIU for anterior stricture management.[7] A recent study looking at national trends continued to show that urethral stricture disease is largely treated by endoscopic urethrotomy or dilation (90.7%) versus urethroplasty (9.3%).[8]

Direct Vision Internal Urethrotomy Technique

The classic technique described by Sachse[6] in 1974 involves making a single 12-o'clock incision into the urethral scar with a cold knife. Variations on this technique have evolved into making 2 or more incisions to release the scar in more than one location. Care must be taken to not extend the incision through the spongiosum but rather just far enough to release the scar to avoid to damage surrounding tissue.

Laser or hot-knife urethrotomy was initiated as an alternative to cold-knife incision to improve outcomes. The types of lasers used include argon, diode, Nd:YAG, and the more common holmium:YAG or holmium laser. Most published studies evaluating the efficacy of laser versus cold-knife urethrotomy indicate no difference in outcomes.[9,10] Although frequently found to decrease operative times, laser urethrotomy is still a higher-cost procedure than traditional cold-knife urethrotomy; thus, cold knife persists as the most commonly performed procedure.[7] Another benefit of cold-knife incision over laser incision is the ability to receive tactile feedback. This feedback allows for precise identification of the release of the contracture associated with the scar (the goal of the procedure) and avoiding an overly aggressive and at times destructive maneuver.

Complications

Postprocedure complications from endoscopic IU may include hematuria, dysuria, urinary tract infection, urinary retention, urinary incontinence, or erectile dysfunction.[11] Overall complication rates are similar between hot- and cold-knife urethrotomy, with the exception of hematuria and urinary retention, which is more common with laser urethrotomy.[11] Reports of erectile dysfunction range from 2.2% to 10.6%, and it is associated with long, dense strictures.[12]

Direct Vision Internal Urethrotomy Outcomes

Literature describing DVIU/dilation outcomes largely consist of case series data with variations in patient population, stricture location and/or length, cause, or primary versus recurrent strictures. Additionally, defining outcomes is limited by the diagnostic criteria used before treatment, the definition of treatment success, patient follow-up, or methods used to determine stricture recurrence.

Although distinct procedures, endoscopic IU and endoscopic UD are deemed nearly equivalent in terms of primary treatment of urethral strictures. Steenkamp and colleagues[13] performed a randomized study comparing stricture-free rates between IU and dilation, which found no statistically significant difference in stricture recurrence rates between IU or UD in a well-matched cohort of 104 and 106 patients, respectively.

Several studies have shown varied success rates of endoscopic incision or dilation based on stricture location and length. In a series of 224 patients with a median 98-month follow-up, Pansadoro and Emiliozzi[3] reported a large discordance in treatment success rates for strictures less than or more than 10 mm in length, 71% versus 18%, respectively.[3] Albers and colleagues[14] reported greater success rates for strictures less than 1 cm; Steenkamp and colleagues[13] also highlighted the importance of size criteria for endoscopic stricture repair, as strictures shorter than 2 cm had a 40% recurrence rate at 12 months, whereas strictures longer than 4 cm had an 80% recurrence rate. In terms of location, penile strictures are associated with the highest recurrence rates after endoscopic dilation or incision, with bulbar strictures being the favored location suitable for this type of repair.[14] Pansadoro and Emiliozzi's[3] series reported similar findings, with recurrence rates after IU of 68% overall, 58% for bulbar, 84% for penile, and 89% for penile bulbar urethral strictures.[3] In addition, treatment success rates of larger-caliber strictures (more than 15 F) are approximately doubled those of narrower lumens, which likely reflects a shallow area of narrowing with minimal spongiofibrosis.[3]

Risks of Repeated Direct Vision Internal Urethrotomy/Dilation

Despite the feasibility of repeated endoscopic treatment of urethral strictures, several studies have reported progressively worse outcomes with each procedure. Although the success of an initial procedure may be 60% to 70%, repeated procedures fail at compounding rates. Heyns and colleagues[15] reported stricture-free rates of 1, 2, or 3 dilations or urethrotomies at 24 months of 60%, 30%, 0%, respectively, and at 48 months rates of 60%, 0%, 0%, respectively. In addition, time to recurrence after a second procedure was dramatically shortened, indicating a limited benefit of a second procedure. There was zero percent success after a third repeat procedure, and this should be viewed as a palliative maneuver.[15] Similarly, Santucci and Eisenberg[16] reported stricture-free rates as low as 6% for a second DVIU and 9%, 0%, 0% for a third, fourth, and fifth. Interestingly, the investigators' reported stricture-free rate for a single procedure was only 8% at 14 months, significantly lower than previously reported success rates. Risks associated with stricture recurrence after dilation or optical urethrotomy include longer (>2 cm) strictures, penile strictures, those occurring after transurethral resection of the prostate (TURP), and those previously treated.[17]

Further risks of repeated urethrotomy or dilation are lower stricture-free rates at the time of definitive urethroplasty.[18] In a more recent analysis of long-term outcomes of urethroplasty, investigators found that prior DVIU was a statistically significant risk factor for treatment failure.[19]

Optimal Indications for Direct Vision Internal Urethrotomy

Based on the aforementioned studies, the ideal patient characteristics for DVIU take into account stricture size, location, caliber, and prior treatment. Prior endoscopic dilation or DVIU seem to be the strongest predictor of treatment failure. Despite this evidence, endoscopic dilation or urethrotomy is the most commonly performed procedure for anterior stricture management.[7,8,20] Therefore, research points to an underutilization of urethroplasty as the definitive repair with a body of literature that demonstrates repeat urethral incision or dilation is not only palliative but can also have a negative effect on stricture-free rates when future urethroplasties are performed (**Table 1**).

Direct Vision Internal Urethrotomy Adjuncts

High recurrence rates for IU led urologists to attempt methods that would increase the durability of this repair. Such approaches included postoperative indwelling urethral catheters, clean intermittent catheterization (CIC), and urethral stenting. More recently, antifibrotic agents have been studied as an alternative to mechanical methods for preventing early scar formation and recurrence.

CIC is suggested in certain patients to maintain patency after a dilation or urethrotomy. Drawbacks to CIC include a risk of minor bleeding in approximately 50% of patients[14] as well as patient dissatisfaction, discomfort, and resistance resulting in a poor quality of life.

Mitomycin C
Mitomycin C (MMC) was first used in IU by Mazdak and colleagues[21] in 2007 as an injection peripheral to the repair site to prevent recurrent scar formation because of its antifibroblast properties.[21] MMC is an antitumor antibiotic isolated from the bacterium

---

Table 1
Risks factors for stricture recurrence after endoscopic treatment

Recurrence Rate	Risk Factor			
	Location	Size	Caliber	Prior DVIU/Dilation
	Penile (84%,[3] 40%[17])	>10 mm (82%[3])	<15F (66%[3])	None (53%,[3] 40%–50%[15])
	Penile bulbar (89%[3])	<10 mm (29%[3])	>15F (31%[3])	1 (100%,[3] 94%,[16] 60%–100%[15])
	Bulbar (58%[3])	>2 cm (59%[17])	—	2 (100%,[15] 91%[16])
	—	<2 cm (26%[17])	—	—

Streptomyces caespitosus, which was first used in urologic surgery as an intravesical therapy to prevent bladder tumor recurrence. It acts as a chemotherapeutic agent by crosslinking DNA and thereby preventing replication.[22] It acts as an antifibroblast agent by preventing fibroblast proliferation and, thereby, scar formation.[23] In nonurological surgeries, MMC is used similarly as a method to prevent scar formation, with frequent application in ophthalmology and otolaryngology.[23,24]

In Mazdak and colleagues'[21] original article, 40 patients with anterior urethral stricture disease were treated with either IU alone or IU with MMC injection. At 6 months, only 10% of strictures recurred in the MCC group compared with 50% treated with DVIU alone.[21] A more recent study evaluated patients with recurrent anterior, posterior, and BNCs with IU and MMC in addition to a daily CIC schedule for 1 month and reported a 75.7% stricture-free rate during the 23-month study period.[25]

Steroid injection

Local steroid injections have also been experimented with as an antiscar adjunctive agent in IU because of its antifibroblast and anticollagen properties. The first known study in the literature included 149 patients randomized to undergo urethrotomy with or without injection of triamcinolone acetonide (TA), with a recurrence rate of 4.3% in the steroid group compared with 19.4% treated without steroid injection.[26] In general, this study reported far higher success rates in both treatment arms than is commonly reported in endoscopic management of urethral stricture disease. Mazdak and colleagues[27] also published their experience using TA injected at the urethrotomy site, with a recurrence rate reduction from 50.0% to 21.7% in 50 patients followed for a mean of 13.7 months with anterior urethral strictures. In contrast, Tabassi and colleagues[28] found a decrease time period to stricture recurrence using TA that was not statistically significant, demonstrating the need to organize larger prospective trials before the use of TA with urethrotomy can be routinely recommended.

POSTERIOR URETHRAL STENOSIS

The posterior urethra includes the membranous and prostatic urethra. It is also vulnerable to stricture formation, most commonly from a traumatic injury (ie, pelvic fracture) or prostate cancer therapy. BNCs are the most common type of stricture formed after radical prostatectomy, whereas radiation-induced strictures commonly manifest in the bulbomembranous urethra.[29]

Bladder Neck Contractures

BNCs are a narrowing of the vesicourethral anastomosis performed during radical prostatectomy. This complication arises in up to 0% to 17.5% of either open or robotic-assisted prostatectomy[30–32] and 1% to 12% of transurethral resection or vaporization of the prostate.[33] The exact causes of BNCs are unknown but related to prior TURP, excessive intraoperative blood loss, the oncologic outcome, urinary extravasation at the vesicourethral anastomosis, or surgical technique of bladder neck reconstruction.[32,34]

Transurethral bladder neck incision

The most commonly performed endoscopic treatment of BNCs is the endoscopic transurethral bladder neck incision (BNI). This technique is generally performed in the same manner as IU for anterior urethral strictures, with a sharp cold-knife or laser/thermal incision performed across the fibrotic scar in 2 to 4 positions. This procedure has a reported success rate of approximately 50% to 70% for primary BNI,[31,33,35] with patients often requiring repeat dilation or incision for recurrence.

Recurrent bladder neck contracture and mitomycin C

In contrast to Mazdak and colleagues'[21] original study, in which patients received MMC during primary repair of an anterior stricture, Vanni and colleagues[36] studied MMC for patients with recurrent BNC after previously failed endoscopic repair. This subgroup population represents a unique challenge as, although recurrent BNCs are uncommon, failure to adequately treat may lead to severe incontinence or obstruction, necessitating an extensive open reconstruction or even a permanent urinary diversion. The investigators performed endoscopic BNIs in a tri or quadrant fashion followed by injection of MMC at each incision site. During a median 12-month follow-up period, 72% of patients achieved a patent bladder neck after only one procedure. Most impressively, 100% of patients who had required an indwelling urethral catheter or regular dilation preoperatively were free of either after the procedure. Another study evaluated a similar procedure with the addition of a strict 1-month CIC schedule. The investigators performed endoscopic BNI with MMC at the incision sites followed by CIC once daily for 1 month postoperatively.[25] Their study also included patients with recurrent stenosis, either anterior or posterior urethral strictures or BNCs. Stricture-free rates were similar between studies, with 72.7% BNCs adequately treated with BNI and MCC plus CIC versus 72.0% with MMC alone. Most recently, Nagpal and colleagues[37] reported a

Table 2
Comparison of endoscopic bladder neck contracture repair techniques

Authors	Technique	Adjuncts	Success after 1 Procedure (%)	Recurrence (%)	Median Follow-up
Primary BNC					
Ramirez et al,[33] 2013, n = 50	BNI, hot knife	—	72	28	12.9 mo
Ishii et al,[39] 2015, n = 10	High-pressure balloon dilation	—	80	20	24.0 mo
Borboroglu et al,[35] 2000, n = 52	BNI or dilation	—	58	42	4.5 y
Recurrent BNC					
Vanni et al,[36] 2011, n = 18	BNI, cold knife	MMC	72	17	12.0 mo
Nagpal et al,[37] 2015, n = 40	BNI, cold knife	MMC	75	25	20.5 mo

large series that demonstrated similar results to previous studies with 75% maintaining a patent bladder neck after one procedure with a 20.5-month follow-up. Although these study results cannot be directly compared, the similar outcomes suggest endoscopic BNI with MMC injection is a promising treatment option for recurrent BNCs (**Table 2**).

Transurethral Balloon Dilation

Transurethral balloon dilation represents an additional, though less commonly used, endoscopic BNC treatment. Older studies describing this technique reported up to a 41% recurrence rate.[38] A more recent study used a high-pressure balloon catheter, dilating the vesicourethral stricture to up to 30 F at 30 atm with a recurrence-free rate of 80% with a 24-month median follow-up.[39] The investigators reported balloon dilation as an alternative to transurethral cold-knife incision that is less invasive and with fewer bleeding complications.

Radiation Induced Stenosis

Pelvic radiation for prostate cancer, including external beam radiotherapy and brachytherapy, is associated with an increased risk for urethral stenosis, with the bulbomembranous urethra cited as the most commonly affected location.[40] The pathophysiology is thought to be progressive microvascular compromise leading to tissue destruction and necrosis. However, the evaluation and management of these radiation-induced strictures (RIS) does not differ from other stricture causes. Although radiation-induced tissue damage would intuitively lead to risk for recurrence, it does not seem to affect stricture recurrence after treatment.[25,33] Endoscopic management and open management of BNC or membranous urethral RIS are more challenging technically, but successful outcomes are possible. As experience with radiation-induced contractures and/or RIS grows, so does the success rates of treatment.[37]

Membranous Urethral Strictures

This situation can be very difficult to manage as patients are obstructed and may or may not be incontinent from a prior TURP procedure, RRP, adjunctive radiation therapy, brachytherapy, or any combination of these. RIS at this location are more challenging to treat but can still have successful outcomes. Endoscopic management is the first-line treatment to relieve obstruction but should be used with caution. Awareness and a discussion with patients preoperatively about the risk of incontinence is critical in situations whereby the internal sphincter located at the bladder neck has been compromised. If endoscopic management fails, patients are offered urethral reconstruction with the discussion that a delayed secondary surgery may be necessary to manage urinary incontinence.

SUMMARY

Urethral stricture disease continues to be a common problem for patients and urologists alike. Endoscopic treatment offers a simple, potentially effective treatment of primary, short, urethral strictures. For patients who recur after endoscopic management, urethral or bladder neck reconstruction should be offered with an experienced urologic reconstructionist familiar with the complexity of the situation and subtleties of the surgery. With the advent of adjunctive antifibrotic agents, durability of endoscopic repair seems to improve but their use requires continued research and longer follow-up to determine their efficacy.

REFERENCES

1. Barbagli G, De Angelis M, Romano G, et al. Long-term follow-up of bulbar end-to-end anastomosis: a retrospective analysis of 153 patients in a single center experience. J Urol 2007;178(6):2470–3.

2. Santucci RA, Mario LA, McAninch JW. Anastomotic urethroplasty for bulbar urethral stricture: analysis of 168 patients. J Urol 2002;167(4):1715–9.

3. Pansodoro V, Emiliozzi P. Internal urethrotomy in the management of anterior urethral strictures: long term follow-up. J Urol 1996;156:73–5.

4. Latini JM, McAninch JW, Brandes SB, et al. SIU/ICUD consultation on urethral strictures: epidemiology, etiology, anatomy, and nomenclature of urethral stenoses, strictures, and pelvic fracture urethral disruption injuries. Urology 2014; 83(3 Suppl):S1–7.

5. Fenton AS, Morey AF, Aviles R, et al. Anterior urethral strictures: etiology and characteristics. Urology 2005;65(6):1055–8.

6. Sachse H. Treatment of urethral stricture: transurethral slit in view using sharp section. Fortschr Med 1974;92(1):12–5 [in German].

7. Ferguson GG, Bullock TL, Anderson RE, et al. Minimally invasive methods for bulbar urethral strictures: a survey of members of the American Urological Association. Urology 2011;78(3):701–6.

8. Buckley JC, Patel N, Wang S, et al. National trends in the management of urethral stricture disease: a 14-year survey of the nationwide inpatient sample. Urol Pract 2016;3(4):315–20.

9. Dutkiewicz SA, Wroblewski M. Comparison of treatment results between holmium laser endourethrotomy and optical internal urethrotomy for urethral stricture. Int Urol Nephrol 2012;44:717–24.

10. Kamp S, Knoll T, Osman MM, et al. Low-power holmium:YAG laser urethrotomy for treatment of urethral strictures: functional outcome and quality of life. J Endourol 2006;20(1):38–41.

11. Jin T, Li H, Jiang LH, et al. Safety and efficacy of laser and cold knife urethrotomy for urethral stricture. Chin Med J (Engl) 2010;123(12):1589–95.

12. Schneider T, Sperling H, Lümmen G, et al. Sachse internal urethrotomy. Is erectile dysfunction a possible complication? Urologe A 2001;40(1):38–41 [in German].

13. Steenkamp JW, Heyns CF, de Kock ML. Internal urethrotomy versus dilation as treatment for male urethral strictures: a prospective, randomized comparison. J Urol 1997;157(1):98–101.

14. Albers P, Fichtner J, Brühl P, et al. Long-term results of internal urethrotomy. J Urol 1996;156(5):1611–4.

15. Heyns CF, Steenkamp JW, De Kock ML, et al. Treatment of male urethral strictures: is repeated dilation or internal urethrotomy useful? J Urol 1998;160(2):356–8.

16. Santucci R, Eisenberg L. Urethrotomy has a much lower success rate than previously reported. J Urol 2010;183(5):1859–62.

17. Zehri AA, Ather MH, Afshan Q. Predictors of recurrence of urethral stricture disease following optical urethrotomy. Int J Surg 2009;7(4):361–4.

18. Roehrborn CG, McConnell JD. Analysis of factors contributing to success or failure of 1-stage urethroplasty for urethral stricture disease. J Urol 1994; 151(4):869–74.

19. Breyer BN, McAninch JW, Whitson JM, et al. Multivariate analysis of risk factors for long-term urethroplasty outcome. J Urol 2010;183(2):613–7.

20. Anger JT, Buckley JC, Santucci RA, et al, Urologic Diseases in America Project. Trends in stricture management among male Medicare beneficiaries: underuse of urethroplasty? Urology 2011;77(2):481–5.

21. Mazdak H, Meshki I, Ghassami F. Effect of mitomycin C on anterior urethral stricture recurrence after internal urethrotomy. Eur Urol 2007;51(4):1089–92 [discussion: 1092].

22. Iyer VN, Szybalski W. Mitomycins and porfiromycin: chemical mechanism of activation and cross-linking of DNA. Science 1964;145(3627):55–8.

23. Jampel HD. Effect of brief exposure to mitomycin C on viability and proliferation of cultured human Tenon's capsule fibroblasts. Ophthalmology 1992;99(9):1471–6.

24. Estrem SA, Vanleeuwen RN. Use of mitomycin C for maintaining myringotomy patency. Otolaryngol Head Neck Surg 2000;122(1):8–10.

25. Farrell MR, Sherer BA, Levine LA. Visual internal urethrotomy with intralesional mitomycin C and short-term clean intermittent catheterization for the management of recurrent urethral strictures and bladder neck contractures. Urology 2015; 85(6):1494–9.

26. Hradec E, Jarolim L, Petrik R. Optical internal urethrotomy for strictures of the male urethra. Effect of local steroid injection. Eur Urol 1981;7(3):165–8.

27. Mazdak H, Izadpanahi MH, Ghalamkari A, et al. Internal urethrotomy and intraurethral submucosal injection of triamcinolone in short bulbar urethral strictures. Int Urol Nephrol 2010;42(3):565–8.

28. Tabassi KT, Yarmohamadi A, Mohammadi S. Triamcinolone injection following internal urethrotomy for treatment of urethral stricture. Urol J 2011;8(2):132–6.

29. Elliott SP, Meng MV, Elkin EP, et al. CaPSURE Investigators. Incidence of urethral stricture after primary treatment for prostate cancer: data From CaPSURE. J Urol 2007;178(2):529–34 [discussion: 534].

30. Breyer BN, Davis CB, Cowan JE, et al. Incidence of bladder neck contracture after robot-assisted laparoscopic and open radical prostatectomy. BJU Int 2010;106(11):1734–8.

31. Popken G, Sommerkamp H, Schultze-Seemann W, et al. Anastomotic stricture after radical prostatectomy. Incidence, findings and treatment. Eur Urol 1998;33(4):382–6.

32. Surya BV, Provet J, Johanson KE, et al. Anastomotic strictures following radical prostatectomy: risk factors and management. J Urol 1990;143(4):755–8.

33. Ramirez D, Zhao LC, Bagrodia A, et al. Deep lateral transurethral incisions for recurrent bladder neck contracture: promising 5-year experience using a standardized approach. Urology 2013;82:1430.

34. Shelfo SW, Obek C, Soloway MS. Update on bladder neck preservation during radical retropubic prostatectomy: impact on pathologic outcome, anastomotic strictures, and incontinence. Urology 1998; 51:73–8.

35. Borboroglu PG, Sands JP, Roberts JL, et al. Risk factors for vesicourethral anastomotic stricture after radical prostatectomy. Urology 2000;56(1): 96–100.

36. Vanni AJ, Zinman LN, Buckley JC. Radial urethrotomy and intralesional mitomycin C for the management of recurrent bladder neck contractures. J Urol 2011;186(1):156–60.

37. Nagpal K, Zinman LN, Lebeis C, et al. Durable results of mitomycin c injection with internal urethrotomy for refractory bladder neck contractures: multi-institutional experience. Urol Pract 2015;2(5): 250–5.

38. Ramchandani P, Banner MP, Berlin JW, et al. Vesicourethral anastomotic strictures after radical prostatectomy: efficacy of transurethral balloon dilation. Radiology 1994;193(2):345–9.

39. Ishii G, Naruoka T, Kasai K, et al. High pressure balloon dilation for vesicourethral anastomotic strictures after radical prostatectomy. BMC Urol 2015;15:62.

40. Sullivan L, Williams SG, Tai KH, et al. Urethral stricture following high dose rate brachytherapy for prostate cancer. Radiother Oncol 2009;91:232–6.

Patient Selection for Urethroplasty Technique
Excision and Primary Reanastomosis Versus Graft

CrossMark

Judith C. Hagedorn, MD, MHS, Bryan B. Voelzke, MD, MS*

KEYWORDS

- Urethral stricture • Urethroplasty • Excision primary anastomosis • Buccal graft

KEY POINTS

- Oral mucosa is the most common and versatile substitution material available today for urethral repair.
- The success rate of excision primary anastomosis has been reported to be excellent (can exceed 90%). It should be considered the optimal treatment of short bulbar urethral strictures.
- If the stricture length, cause, and/or patient characteristics necessitate substitution urethroplasty, the surgeon can choose from a variety of techniques for a bulbar urethral stricture.
- Patients should be surgically managed based on their individual circumstances. Surgeons should choose a familiar surgical approach that is based on a patient's clinical characteristics.

INTRODUCTION

It is difficult to make best clinical practice recommendations on the management of urethral stricture disease. There is a lack of evidence to allow definitive recommendations regarding which circumstances to perform a particular urethroplasty technique. The management of bulbar urethral stricture disease remains a source of controversy and depends on the characteristics of the urethral stricture as well as patient characteristics and surgeon preference. Among bulbar urethral strictures, a buccal graft can be used or the urethra can be excised and primarily reanastomosed. These 2 options do not exist in the penile urethra, because excision and primary anastomosis of the urethra is contraindicated. As such, the aim of this review is to describe the various surgical techniques of bulbar urethral stricture surgery with associated outcomes and complications, with emphasis on individualized therapy.

Excision and primary reanastomosis (EPA) of a bulbar urethral stricture is the simplest surgical option; however, certain urethral strictures and patient characteristics demand the use of a graft or flap substitution. Several different grafts have been described, including penile skin, scrotal skin, extragenital skin, bladder mucosa, colonic mucosa and buccal mucosa. Initially, skin grafts or flaps were used for substitution bulbar urethroplasty; however, buccal mucosa grafts (BMGs) have since replaced skin grafts.[1] The oral mucosa graft urethroplasty was first described by the Russian surgeon Kirill Sapezhko in 1890.[2] Approximately 50 years later buccal mucosa was described for urethral repair, and another

Conflicts of Interest: None.
Disclosures: None for either author.
Department of Urology, Harborview Medical Center, University of Washington, Box 359868, 325 9th Avenue, Seattle, WA 98104, USA
* Corresponding author.
E-mail address: voelzke@uw.edu

urologic.theclinics.com

40 years passed before this technique could be found in the literature again.[3,4] Nowadays it is the most common graft used in urethral reconstruction.

A recent multi-institutional study on 466 patients found higher complication and restricture rates with skin flaps versus BMG for long strictures.[5] The preference for buccal mucosa is due to its ease of harvest, reliable take, and few donor site complications; hence, it can be considered the gold standard for substitution urethroplasty.[6,7] The BMG has a dense capillary network in the submucosa. Through imbibition and inosculation from the graft bed, BMGs are incorporated into the surrounding tissue.[8] Because the BMG initially depends on nutrients and revascularization from the surrounding tissue, it is important to provide a healthy and vascularized recipient site for successful graft take.

ANATOMIC CONSIDERATIONS

To make appropriate reconstructive decisions, it is mandatory to understand the anatomy of the bulbar urethra that is positioned between the distal penile urethra and more proximal membranous urethra. The bulbar urethra is part of the anterior urethra and is surrounded by vascularized corpus spongiosum that is covered ventrally by the bulbo-spongiosus muscle.[9] At the bulbar urethra, the lumen is located dorsally and not centrally, rendering the corpus spongiosum thick on the ventral surface and thin on the dorsal surface (**Fig. 1**). The corpus spongiosum serves as a vascularized mechanical support for substitution grafts, especially with ventral grafting. The spongiosum may not be sufficient for mechanical support, which can lead to sacculation if a ventral graft is used.[10]

The internal pudendal artery is the primary source of blood supply to the penis. The internal pudendal artery branches to the inferior rectal, posterior scrotal, and penile arteries. The penile artery subsequently branches into the dorsal, bulbar, and cavernosal arteries (**Fig. 2**). The bulbar urethra travels in the deep perineal space to supply the corpus spongiosum and urethra. The bulbar artery connects to the dorsal penile artery at the glans penis, allowing the urethra to get antegrade and retrograde blood supply. The dorsal penile artery runs along the dorsum of the penis and supplies the penile skin, fascia, and glans penis. As the dorsal artery travels distally along the penis, circumflex arteries periodically branch

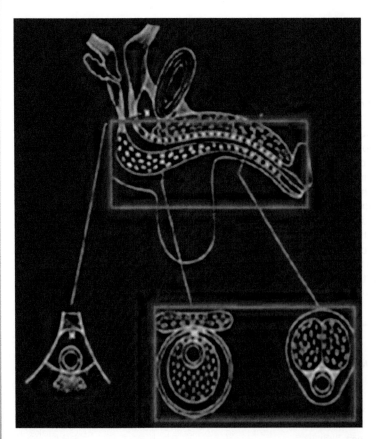

Fig. 1. Cross-section of urethra at the membranous (*left line*), bulbar (*middle line*), and penile (*right line*) urethra. The bulbar urethra has abundant ventral corpus spongiosum resulting in the urethral lumen being more dorsally located. The penile urethra has limited ventral corpus spongiosum. The paired corpora cavernosa are dorsal (posterior) to the penile urethra. (*From* Turner-Warwick R. Urethral stricture surgery. In: Mundy AR, editor. Current operative surgery: urology. London: W.B. Saunders; 1988. p. 160–218; with permission.)

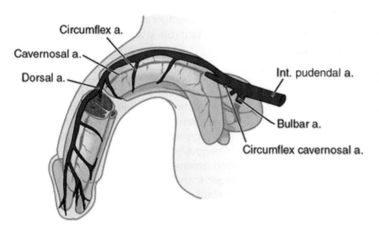

Fig. 2. Penile arterial blood supply. a., artery; Int, internal. (*From* Keegan KA, Penson DF. Vasculogenic erectile function. In: Creagor MA, Beckman JA, Loscalzo J, editors. Vascular medicine: a companion to Braunwald's heart disease. Philadelphia: Elsevier Saunders; 2013. p. 343; with permission.)

off laterally to supply the corpus spongiosum. The cavernosal artery is an end artery that supplies the corpus cavernosum. It is critical to understand the implications of penile dissection and urethral mobilization. If the urethra is mobilized off the corpora cavernosa (as with a dorsal onlay BMG urethroplasty or after urethral mobilization for EPA urethroplasty), the circumflex arterial supply can be impaired. Likewise, transection of the bulbar urethra and spongiosum (as with an EPA or augmented urethroplasty) can result in loss of antegrade blood flow to the urethra distal to the transection. Fortunately, retrograde blood flow from the dorsal penile artery and circumflex blood vessels can provide arterial blood supply. Excessive mobilization of the penile urethra, a hypospadiac deformity, and distal spongiofibrosis compromise the retrograde flow derived from the distal collaterals and may impair graft take or lead to stricture recurrence secondary to ischemia.

Several techniques have been described to preserve optimal blood supply. Jordan and colleagues[11] have proposed a vessel-sparing approach to EPA urethral reconstruction to preserve the best vascularity. They preserved the bulbar arteries by dissecting them off the urethra ventrally and left the ventral corpus spongiosum intact (**Fig. 3**). Even though they could not show superior outcomes concerning stricture patency, they were able to demonstrate that preservation of the blood supply was possible and may be considered as the preferred technique for patients with compromised vascularity and/or who might need adjuvant urethral surgery in the future (ie, artificial urinary sphincter).

Kulkarni and colleagues[12] described the successful results of a 1-sided dorsal onlay graft technique, avoiding extensive, circumferential dissection of the urethra. It is a modification to the traditional dorsal onlay technique that involves a circumferential mobilization of the bulbar urethra. As a modification

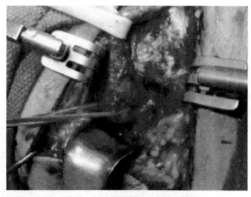
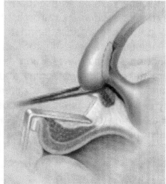

Fig. 3. Vessel loop is placed around bulbar vessel for bulbar artery-sparing surgery (*left*). Dotted line: the dorsal urethrotomy is made without injury to the bulbar vessels, leaving the ventral spongiosum intact (*right*). (*From* Jordan GH, Eltahawy EA, Virasoro R. The technique of vessel sparing excision and primary anastomosis for proximal bulbous urethral reconstruction. J Urol 2007;177(5):1800; with permission.)

of this technique, they proposed to dissect only on 1 side of the urethra, preserving the lateral circumflex blood supply, central tendon of the perineum, and the bulbospongiosus muscle. The bulbospongiosus muscle can be split vertically when the stricture involves the bulbar urethra. The dorsal urethral dissection is carried out just past the dorsal midline, to make the dorsal urethrotomy and to quilt the buccal graft to the tunica albuginea overlying the corpora cavernosa.[12] The Heineke-Mikulicz repair was described as an alternative to an EPA for very short strictures of less than or equal to 1 cm, with a wide caliber and minimal fibrosis. The urethra is not transected as with a traditional EPA, but a longitudinal stricturotomy is made and closed transversely, keeping the retrograde blood flow intact.[13]

Innervation of the bulbar urethra and bulbospongiosus muscle is also important for surgical outcomes. Previous research has revealed that branches of the perineal nerve do extend into the bulbospongiosus muscle.[14,15] Therefore, impaired nerve function from a bulbar urethroplasty with the standard approach of transection of the bulbospongiosus muscle potentially explains the loss of the bulbar contractions needed for efficient semen emission and could lead to postvoid dribbling. A bulbospongiosus muscle-sparing approach for the bulbar urethroplasty has been described, leaving the lateral muscle attachments and central tendon intact and thereby preserving the perineal nerves.[16] None of the patients in a comparative study of the impact of bulbospongiosus muscle-sparing surgery to transection of this muscle reported a decreased force of semen emission, and none complained of postvoid dribbling. With division of the bulbospongiosus muscle, the investigators reported sluggish ejaculation in 20% and postvoid dribbling in 50%.[16] A randomized study of the effect of bulbospongiosus muscle transection versus preservation during bulbar urethroplasty was subsequently performed in an attempt to replicate these findings. The investigators did not note an impact on ejaculatory function or postvoid dribbling.[17] This study was small and may have had limited power to assess a difference. Further study is needed to assess if bulbospongiosus muscle-sparing surgery provides benefit to any particular patient populations.

BULBAR URETHRAL STRICTURE CHARACTERISTICS

Anatomic considerations are the cornerstone for all surgical interventions; however, the presenting features of the stricture and patient characteristics play an important role in surgical decision making.

Stricture Length

Not all bulbar urethral strictures are the same and much of the treatment decision depends on length and etiology. Stricture length is one of the characteristics that has a great impact on reconstruction choice. Previously, short strictures of 1 cm were considered amenable to an EPA, whereas strictures longer than 1 cm were traditionally treated with substitution urethroplasty.[18] The rationale was to avoid tension on the anastomosis leading to stricture recurrence and possible penile curvature and shortening. With passage of time, the accepted limits to EPA urethroplasty have expanded. Morey and McAninch[19] proposed a stricture length of 2.5 cm to be considered for EPA, and thereafter several studies have reported acceptable outcomes with excision of isolated bulbar strictures up to 4.5 cm.[19–21]

It is theorized that more proximal bulbar urethral strictures can be excised in longer lengths without jeopardizing the antegrade blood flow to the most distally transected portion of the urethra; however, there is a limit to the length of urethra that can be safely transected, because unintended consequences can occur.[22] Tension on the reanastomosed urethra after EPA repair can lead to penile curvature after excessive urethral excision.[23] When performing an EPA, the entire stricture needs to be excised, leaving only healthy urethra for planned reanastomosis (**Fig. 4**). A tension-free anastomosis can usually be achieved, and urethral mobilization to the penoscrotal junction can be used to enable a tension-free anastomosis. Only rarely is it necessary to split the corporal bodies to achieve tension-free urethral continuity. Using these techniques, EPA repair can be highly successful with a low complication rate.[24] The Société Internationale d'Urologie with the International Consultation on Urological Diseases published a literature review on primary anastomosis anterior urethroplasty and reported a success rate of 93.8% and a negligible effect on sexual function.[24]

Although EPA urethroplasty has the highest success rate for bulbar strictures, substitution urethroplasty with buccal mucosa has a considerably high success rate as well, approximately 85% to 90%.[25,26] In contrast to EPA repair, substitution urethroplasty has a steady failure rate that increases over the years. Previous reports examining long-term success at 5-year, 10-year, and 15-year periods noted restricture results that were 12%, 13%, and

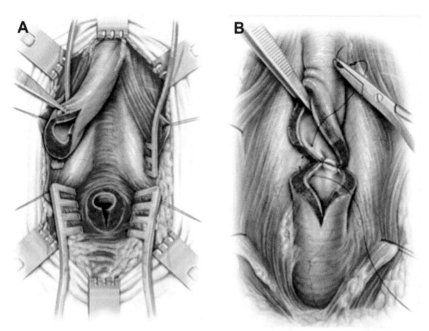

Fig. 4. Excision and primary anastomosis. Urethra following excision of stricture (A). Primary anastomosis of urethral ends following excision of urethral stricture (B). (*From* Mundy AR. Surgical atlas anastomotic urethroplasty. BJU Int 2005;96:927–8; with permission.)

14% for anastomotic repairs and 21%, 31%, and 58% for substitution urethroplasty, respectively.[27]

When the urethral stricture is too long for an EPA repair, the options then include stricture incision with substitution graft onlay (ventral, dorsal or lateral), graft inlay (Asopa or Palminteri), or an excision with an augmented roof strip (**Figs. 5–8**). Before the introduction of the dorsal onlay technique by Barbagli in 1996,[28] bulbar strictures were traditionally repaired with a ventral stricturotomy and graft onlay (see **Fig. 5**). The dorsal onlay has gained widespread acceptance with suggested benefits of less bleeding from the thinner dorsal spongiosum and more stable fixation of the graft to the corpora cavernosa, providing a nourishing graft bed, the potential for proximal and distal extension of the urethrotomy, and theoretically limited sacculation (see **Fig. 6**).[26,29] Nevertheless, the ventral onlay should be considered for proximal bulbar strictures when there is limited spongiofibrosis, because the ventral approach can provide better exposure.[3] Additionally, when dealing with radiation-induced strictures or particularly high-risk patients with long strictures, a ventral BMG maybe the best choice, because it can be supported by a gracilis muscle flap, giving the BMG a healthy graft bed.[30] The

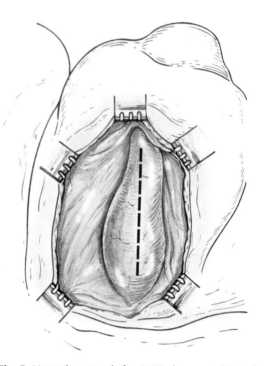

Fig. 5. Ventral approach for BMG placement (*dotted line* denotes planned incision along midline of ventral urethra). (*From* Mangera A, Patterson JM, Chapple CR. A systematic review of graft augmentation urethroplasty techniques for the treatment of anterior urethral strictures. Eur Urol 2011;59(5):798; with permission.)

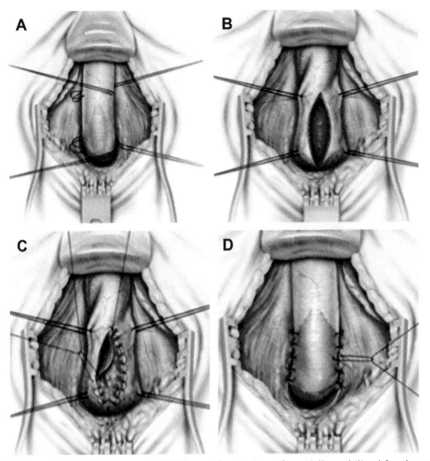

Fig. 6. Dorsal approach for BMG placement. (*A*) The urethra is circumferentially mobilized for the entire length of the stricture an approximately 1.5 cm beyond the stricture distally and proximally. (*B*) The urethra is rotated 180°. The urethrotomy is made on the dorsal aspect and stay sutures are placed. (*C*) The BMG sutured into place. (*D*) The urethra and corpus spongiosum are sutured to the tunica albuginea, giving support to the urethral reconstruction. (*From* Riechardt S, Pfalzgraf D, Dahlem R, et al. Focus on details dorsal buccal mucosa inlay for penile urethroplasty. BJU Int 2009;103:1445–6; with permission.)

lateral onlay was described in 2005 and theorized that it may be useful for patients who would have significant bleeding with the ventral approach or for patients whose erectile function may be adversely affected by dorsal dissection (see **Fig. 7**).[31] The lateral approach has only been described in a handful of patients and is used infrequently, likely because of a lack of advantage over the other onlay techniques.

The dorsal and ventral approaches have been compared in the literature. A literature review of graft augmentation urethroplasty noted similar success rates for the ventral and dorsal approach (88.84% vs 88.37%); however, these statements should not be taken as fact.[26] One randomized controlled trial of dorsal versus ventral BMG does exist that included 40 patients in each group.[32] The efficacy and complications rates were equal in the 2 groups at 12 months'

follow-up. The methods section of the randomized controlled trial did not have details about the statistical power of the study; therefore, the possibility that no difference between ventral and dorsal onlay was detected due to a small number of patients that were randomized cannot be excluded. The Société Internationale d'Urologie with the International Consultation on Urological Diseases has also published a systemic review on anterior urethral stricture disease using substitution urethroplasty and concluded that there is no significant difference in outcome between the ventral, lateral, dorsal, or combined approach.[33] A statistically powered randomized study of dorsal versus ventral surgery has never been performed, precluding the ability to compare dorsal and ventral BMG repairs. Comparisons of success between dorsal and ventral BMG repairs are limited by selection bias,

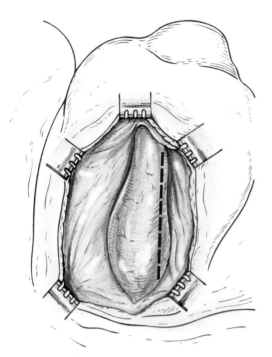

Fig. 7. Lateral approach for BMG placement (*dotted line* denotes planned incision along lateral aspect of ventral urethra). (*From* Mangera A, Patterson JM, Chapple CR. A systematic review of graft augmentation urethroplasty techniques for the treatment of anterior urethral strictures. Eur Urol 2011;59(5):798; with permission.)

because most reconstructive surgeons opt for a dorsal onlay BMG instead of ventral BMG surgery if there is significant spongiofibrosis. Until such studies are performed, comparison of ventral and dorsal BMG repairs should be done with caution.

An alternative inlay procedure has been described by Asopa and colleagues[34] with a reported success rate of 87%. A ventral urethrotomy is made, followed by incision of the dorsal urethra down to the tunica albuginea, where the BMG is placed (see **Fig. 8**). Palminteri and colleagues[35] added a ventral onlay to the dorsal inlay and reported a similar success rate of 89% with a mean follow-up of 22 months. A combined ventral and dorsal BMG has also been described for the repair of long obliterative strictures without incision of the ventral corpus spongiosum. This approach may be considered in patients with a history of hypospadias or distal urethral surgery, with a compromised retrograde blood flow where urethral transection should be avoided.[36] The urethra is mobilized and a ventral BMG is placed onto the spongiosum after removal of a ventral mucosal strip and a dorsal graft is placed onto the corpora cavernosa.

Stricture Etiology

Stricture etiology can be difficult to discern, because an idiopathic etiology is most commonly noted in the modern literature. Stricture etiology can differ based on geographic location, as reported in a recent article examining stricture demographics among patients from the United States, Italy, and India.[37] Idiopathic and iatrogenic strictures were more common among patients from the United States and Italy, whereas traumatic strictures were most common among patients from India. Data from the United States and Italy also supported idiopathic and iatrogenic strictures as most common followed by traumatic and lichen sclerosus strictures as less common.[38] When a cause is known, this knowledge should have an impact on the decision regarding surgical technique. For example, the bulbomembranous stricture that occurs after blunt pelvic fracture injury is best treated by EPA repair. These injuries result in a distraction defect and complete obliteration of the urethral lumen. As such, an anastomotic urethroplasty after complete excision of the scar tissue is the preferred surgery due to

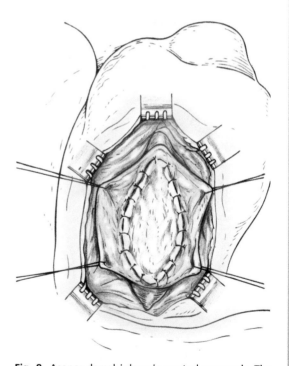

Fig. 8. Asopa: dorsal inlay via ventral approach. The ventral corpus spongiosum is opened and the dorsal urethral plate is incised. The BMG is sewn in dorsally and the ventral corpus spongiosum is closed. (*From* Mangera A, Patterson JM, Chapple CR. A systematic review of graft augmentation urethroplasty techniques for the treatment of anterior urethral strictures. Eur Urol 2011;59(5):799; with permission.)

high success with durable outcomes.[27] Similarly, perineal straddle injuries can result in varying degrees of spongiofibrosis. When associated with severe spongiofibrosis and limited urethral lumen, an EPA repair should be strongly considered. In some cases, the obliterated urethral segment exists in conjunction with a nonobliterated but symptomatic urethral stricture that is greater than 2 cm to 3 cm. In such a setting, an EPA alone may not be possible due to stricture length. For these strictures, the augmented anastomotic approach is useful, excising and performing an anastomosis on 1 side of the urethra, while placing a BMG in the remaining segment with a relatively better caliber (**Fig. 9**).[1] In contrast, strictures due to lichen sclerosis most primarily affect the penile urethra and tend to be longer. EPA urethroplasty is contraindicated in the penile urethra, and substitution urethroplasty is a recognized surgical approach.[27,39] For long strictures (>2–3 cm) that do not allow EPA repair, 1-stage substitution urethroplasty may not be possible if the urethral plate is not wide enough. In such situations, staged repair using BMG should be considered.[40]

Concerning lichen sclerosus, the success rate of urethral repair is significantly lower for patients with the skin disease than without the inflammatory condition. Erickson and colleagues[39] from the Trauma and Urologic Reconstruction Network of Surgeons analyzed strictures of 1151 men from their multi-institutional database. Patients with lichen sclerosis had on average longer strictures, mostly involving the penile urethra and rarely the bulbar urethra alone. None of the lichen sclerosus strictures was treated with an EPA repair; rather, substitution urethroplasty was primarily used. Substitution urethoplasty had a significantly lower success rate than strictures due to other causes (82% vs 92%). A significantly higher rate of chronic, systemic inflammatory conditions, such as hypertension, diabetes, and obesity, was noted in the lichen sclerosus patients compared with patients without the condition.[39]

PATIENT CHARACTERISTICS

Surgical treatment of bulbar strictures is mostly guided by the presenting features of the stricture, such as etiology, degree of spongiofibrosis, length, and location. Despite this, patient characteristics are an equally important risk factor affecting surgical success. In a large series of 443 patients who underwent urethroplasty, risk factors affecting failure were retrospectively examined.[41] Smoking, previous DVIU, and prior urethroplasty were independent predictors of urethroplasty failure. Diabetes mellitus trended toward significance. Although diabetes cannot be altered in a majority of circumstances and obesity management can be challenging for some

A   B

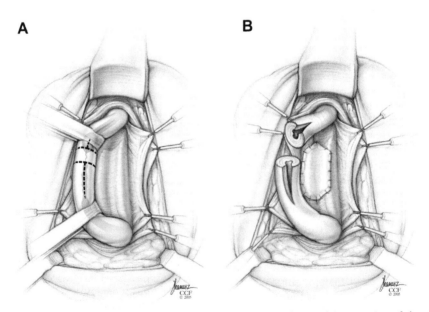

Fig. 9. Augmented urethroplasty. From (*A*) Dotted lines mark excision of most dense portion of the stricture and dorsal urethrotomy into healthy urethra proximally and distally. (*B*) The buccoal mucosa graft is quilted onto the corpora cavernosa tunica albuginea and the native urethra is anastomosed as a roof strip and fixed to the graft laterally. (*From* Abouassaly R, Angermeier KW. Augmented anastomotic urethroplasty. J Urol 177;6:2212; with permission.)

patients, the reconstructive urologist can make an impact on a patient's smoking status. The negative impact of smoking has been conclusively documented in the general surgery literature.[42,43] Surgeons should counsel patients, provide information and resources for smoking cessation, and convey that smoking cessation can have a positive impact on surgical success.

The finding that previous DVIU may contribute to treatment failure is not novel but remains controversial. Some studies have shown that urethroplasty outcomes are worse for patients who have had failed urethrotomy before the definite repair.[44–46] For both substitution urethroplasty and anastomotic repair, the success for a primary repair is higher than for an urethroplasty after prior surgical manipulation, such as dilation or DIVU.[44–46] In contrast, others have reported that the success rate was not different for patients with prior failed urethrotomy versus patients who underwent a primary urethral repair without previous surgical intervention (87% vs 85%).[47] Similar success rates were noted for both an anastomotic repair and a substitution urethroplasty. Even though the literature does not provide definite data, most investigators would argue that 1 attempt at DVIU may be attempted for a short, wide-caliber bulbar stricture; however, if unsuccessful, further manipulation should be avoided in lieu of open urethral reconstruction if the patient is a surgical candidate.

COMPLICATIONS

Not only is it important to make the correct reconstructive choice based on the stricture etiology and length as well as patient characteristics but also surgeons must be aware of complications inherent in each reconstructive technique. The complication profile differs between anastomotic and substitution urethroplasty.[27] Penile curvature is possible after EPA urethroplasty when a longer segment of urethra is excised. This results in more tension with the anastomosis and a greater likelihood for subsequent penile curvature. Some investigators report no complications with EPA urethroplasty if chosen for the correct bulbar stricture, namely less than 3 cm in length, which prevents potential curvature or shortening of the penis.[22]

After bulbar urethroplasty, a worrisome complication that has been reported is new onset of erectile dysfunction. Theoretically, the cavernous nerves may be damaged where they emerge from the pelvic floor close to the proximal bulbar urethra.[48] This loss of erectile function is mostly seen with EPA and not substitution urethroplasty.[49] A vast majority of patients recover previous sexual function within 6 months of surgery; hence, observation of any degree of erectile dysfunction is prudent in the early postoperative period.[50,51] This was confirmed by a meta-analysis on de novo erectile dysfunction after anterior urethroplasty. This systematic review of the literature reported the risk of de novo erectile dysfunction as approximately 1%, which resolves in many cases within the first year after surgery. There was no significant association between the number of failed previous interventions, including direct vision internal urethrotomy (DVIU), urethral dilation, or urethroplasty, to the onset of erectile dysfunction after anterior urethroplasty.[52] One study compares urethroplasty techniques and determined that the factor influencing sexual function after surgery is stricture length and not the specific surgical procedure. Men with strictures close to 7 cm reported worse erectile function than men with strictures up to approximately 5 cm.[53] In addition, when the stricture is due to pelvic trauma, erectile dysfunction is related to the severity of the original injury and not the stricture repair.[54]

Graft urethral reconstruction comes with more potential complications than the EPA repair. The additional complications reported for substitution urethroplasty are dependent on the graft location. The ventral approach is thought of as technically easier,[55] but it carries the risk of sacculation because the graft is only supported by the spongiosum and not the tunica albuginea and underlying erectile tissue as it is with the dorsal placement.[56,57] In addition, the ventral graft is closer to the skin and, therefore, a urethrocutaneous fistula can rarely occur.[27] The dorsal onlay does not carry these risks, but the dissection and graft placement are technically more challenging. The lateral approach and the inlay procedures (described previously) have not been investigated with long enough follow-up to make a statement about differences in complications.

SUMMARY

In conclusion, appropriate patient selection for EPA versus BMG urethroplasty depends mainly on stricture length, location, and etiology. The optimal treatment of bulbar strictures is an EPA, with a very high and lasting success rate. If a tension-free anastomosis cannot be achieved due to the length of the diseased urethral segment, or it is deemed inappropriate due to the stricture etiology or patient characteristics, substitution is used with potential excision of the completely obliterated lumen. For substitution, a BMG is the most commonly used and versatile graft material. To achieve the best outcomes, anatomic principals must be considered to provide the best blood supply to the anastomosis and/or graft and patients should be counseled regarding optimization of their medical health.

REFERENCES

1. Andrich DE, Mundy AR. What is the best technique for urethroplasty? Eur Urol 2008;54(5):1031–41.
2. Korneyev I, Ilyin D, Schultheiss D, et al. The first oral mucosal graft urethroplasty was carried out in the 19th century: the pioneering experience of Kirill Sapezhko (1857-1928). Eur Urol 2012;62(4):624–7.
3. Patterson JM, Chapple CR. Surgical techniques in substitution urethroplasty using buccal mucosa for the treatment of anterior urethral strictures. Eur Urol 2008;53(6):1162–71.
4. Humby GA. One-stage operation for hypospadias. Br J Surg 1941;(29):84–92.
5. Warner JN, Malkawi I, Dhradkeh M, et al. A Multi-institutional evaluation of the management and outcomes of long-segment urethral strictures. Urology 2015;85(6):1483–7.
6. Markiewicz MR, Lukose MA, Margarone JE 3rd, et al. The oral mucosa graft: a systematic review. J Urol 2007;178(2):387–94.
7. Bhargava S, Chapple CR. Buccal mucosal urethroplasty: is it the new gold standard? BJU Int 2004;93(9):1191–3.
8. Duckett JW, Coplen D, Ewalt D, et al. Buccal mucosal urethral replacement. J Urol 1995;153(5):1660–3.
9. Mundy A. Male urethra. In: Standring S, editor. Gray's anatomy. Edinburgh (IN): Elsevier; 2005. p. 1295–8.
10. Bhandari M, Dubey D, Verma BS. Dorsal or ventral placement of the preputial/penile skin onlay flap for anterior urethral strictures:does it make a difference? BJU Int 2001;88(1):39–43.
11. Jordan GH, Eltahawy EA, Virasoro R. The technique of vessel sparing excision and primary anastomosis for proximal bulbous urethral reconstruction. J Urol 2007;177(5):1799–802.
12. Kulkarni S, Barbagli G, Sansalone S, et al. One-sided anterior urethroplasty: a new dorsal onlay graft technique. BJU Int 2009;104(8):1150–5.
13. Lumen N, Hoebeke P, Oosterlinck W. Ventral longitudinal stricturotomy and transversal closure: the Heineke-Mikulicz principle in urethroplasty. Urology 2010;76(6):1478–82.
14. Yang CC, Bradley WE. Somatic innervation of the human bulbocavernosus muscle. Clin Neurophysiol 1999;110(3):412–8.
15. Yucel S, Baskin LS. Neuroanatomy of the male urethra and perineum. BJU Int 2003;92(6):624–30.
16. Barbagli G, De Stefani S, Annino F, et al. Muscle- and nerve-sparing bulbar urethroplasty: a new technique. Eur Urol 2008;54(2):335–43.
17. Fredrick A, Erickson B, Stensland K, et al. Critical analysis of Bulbospongiosus sparing bulbar urethroplasty on ejaculatory function and post-void dribbling. AUA annual meeting, San Diego, CA, May 9, 2016.
18. Webster GD, Koefoot RB, Sihelnik SA. Urethroplasty management in 100 cases of urethral stricture: a rationale for procedure selection. J Urol 1985;134(5):892–8.
19. Morey AF, McAninch JW. Sonographic staging of anterior urethral strictures. J Urol 2000;163(4):1070–5.
20. Santucci RA, Mario LA, McAninch JW. Anastomotic urethroplasty for bulbar urethral stricture: analysis of 168 patients. J Urol 2002;167(4):1715–9.
21. Eltahawy EA, Virasoro R, Schlossberg SM, et al. Long-term followup for excision and primary anastomosis for anterior urethral strictures. J Urol 2007;177(5):1803–6.
22. Micheli E, Ranieri A, Peracchia G, et al. End-to-end urethroplasty: long-term results. BJU Int 2002;90(1):68–71.
23. Palminteri E, Franco G, Berdondini E, et al. Anterior urethroplasty and effects on sexual life: which is the best technique? Minerva Urol Nefrol 2010;62(4):371–6.
24. Morey AF, Watkin N, Shenfeld O, et al. SIU/ICUD consultation on urethral strictures: anterior urethra–primary anastomosis. Urology 2014;83(3 Suppl):S23–6.
25. Bugeja S, Andrich DE, Mundy AR. Non-transecting bulbar urethroplasty. Transl Androl Urol 2015;4(1):41–50.
26. Mangera A, Patterson JM, Chapple CR. A systematic review of graft augmentation urethroplasty techniques for the treatment of anterior urethral strictures. Eur Urol 2011;59(5):797–814.
27. Andrich DE, Dunglison N, Greenwell TJ, et al. The long-term results of urethroplasty. J Urol 2003;170(1):90–2.
28. Barbagli G, Selli C, Tosto A, et al. Dorsal free graft urethroplasty. J Urol 1996;155(1):123–6.
29. Venkatesan K, Blakely S, Nikolavsky D. Surgical repair of bulbar urethral strictures: advantages of ventral, dorsal, and lateral approaches and when to choose them. Adv Urol 2015;2015:397936.
30. Palmer DA, Buckley JC, Zinman LN, et al. Urethroplasty for high risk, long segment urethral strictures with ventral buccal mucosa graft and gracilis muscle flap. J Urol 2015;193(3):902–5.
31. Barbagli G, Palminteri E, Guazzoni G, et al. Bulbar urethroplasty using buccal mucosa grafts placed on the ventral, dorsal or lateral surface of the urethra: are results affected by the surgical technique? J Urol 2005;174(3):955–7 [discussion: 957–8].

32. Vasudeva P, Nanda B, Kumar A, et al. Dorsal versus ventral onlay buccal mucosal graft urethroplasty for long-segment bulbar urethral stricture: a prospective randomized study. Int J Urol 2015;22(10): 967–71.

33. Chapple C, Andrich D, Atala A, et al. SIU/ICUD Consultation on Urethral Strictures: the management of anterior urethral stricture disease using substitution urethroplasty. Urology 2014; 83(3 Suppl):S31–47.

34. Asopa HS, Garg M, Singhal GG, et al. Dorsal free graft urethroplasty for urethral stricture by ventral sagittal urethrotomy approach. Urology 2001;58(5): 657–9.

35. Palminteri E, Manzoni G, Berdondini E, et al. Combined dorsal plus ventral double buccal mucosa graft in bulbar urethral reconstruction. Eur Urol 2008;53(1):81–9.

36. Gelman J, Siegel JA. Ventral and dorsal buccal grafting for 1-stage repair of complex anterior urethral strictures. Urology 2014;83(6):1418–22.

37. Alwaal A, Blaschko SD, McAninch JW, et al. Epidemiology of urethral strictures. Transl Androl Urol 2014;3(2):209–13.

38. Stein DM, Thum DJ, Barbagli G, et al. A geographic analysis of male urethral stricture aetiology and location. BJU Int 2013;112(6):830–4.

39. Erickson BA, Elliott SP, Myers JB, et al. Understanding the relationship between chronic systemic disease and lichen sclerosus urethral strictures. J Urol 2016;195(2):363–8.

40. Palminteri E, Brandes SB, Djordjevic M. Urethral reconstruction in lichen sclerosus. Curr Opin Urol 2012;22(6):478–83.

41. Breyer BN, McAninch JW, Whitson JM, et al. Multivariate analysis of risk factors for long-term urethroplasty outcome. J Urol 2010;183(2):613–7.

42. Khullar D, Maa J. The impact of smoking on surgical outcomes. J Am Coll Surg 2012;215(3):418–26.

43. Sørensen LT, Jørgensen T. Short-term pre-operative smoking cessation intervention does not affect postoperative complications in colorectal surgery: a randomized clinical trial. Colorectal Dis 2003; 5(4):347–52.

44. Roehrborn CG, McConnell JD. Analysis of factors contributing to success or failure of 1-stage urethroplasty for urethral stricture disease. J Urol 1994; 151(4):869–74.

45. de la Rosette JJ, de Vries JD, Lock MT, et al. Urethroplasty using the pedicled island flap technique in complicated urethral strictures. J Urol 1991; 146(1):40–2.

46. Martinez-Pineiro JA, Carcamo P, Garcia Matres MJ, et al. Excision and anastomotic repair for urethral stricture disease: experience with 150 cases. Eur Urol 1997;32(4):433–41.

47. Barbagli G, Palminteri E, Lazzeri M, et al. Long-term outcome of urethroplasty after failed urethrotomy versus primary repair. J Urol 2001;165(6 Pt 1): 1918–9.

48. Lue TF, Zeineh SJ, Schmidt RA, et al. Neuroanatomy of penile erection: its relevance to iatrogenic impotence. J Urol 1984;131(2):273–80.

49. Yuri P, Wahyudi I, Rodjani A. Comparison between end-to-end anastomosis graft in short segment bulbar urethral stricture: a meta-analysis study. Acta Med Indones 2016;48(1):17–27.

50. Erickson BA, Granieri MA, Meeks JJ, et al. Prospective analysis of erectile dysfunction after anterior urethroplasty: incidence and recovery of function. J Urol 2010;183(2):657–61.

51. Beysens M, Palminteri E, Oosterlinck W, et al. Anastomotic repair versus free graft urethroplasty for bulbar strictures: a focus on the impact on sexual function. Adv Urol 2015;2015:912438.

52. Blaschko SD, Sanford MT, Cinman NM, et al. De novo erectile dysfunction after anterior urethroplasty: a systematic review and meta-analysis. BJU Int 2013;112(5):655–63.

53. Coursey JW, Morey AF, McAninch JW, et al. Erectile function after anterior urethroplasty. J Urol 2001; 166(6):2273–6.

54. El-Assmy A, Harraz AM, Benhassan M, et al. Erectile function after anastomotic urethroplasty for pelvic fracture urethral injuries. Int J Impot Res 2016;28: 139–42.

55. Barbagli G, Montorsi F, Guazzoni G, et al. Ventral oral mucosal onlay graft urethroplasty in nontraumatic bulbar urethral strictures: surgical technique and multivariable analysis of results in 214 patients. Eur Urol 2013;64(3):440–7.

56. Brigman JA, Deture FA. Giant urethral diverticulum after free full thickness skin graft urethroplasty. J Urol 1979;121(4):523–4.

57. Iselin CE, Webster GD. Dorsal onlay graft urethroplasty for repair of bulbar urethral stricture. J Urol 1999;161(3):815–8.

Graft Use in Bulbar Urethroplasty

Mya E. Levy, MD, Sean P. Elliott, MD, MS*

KEYWORDS

- Buccal graft • Urethroplasty • Ventral onlay • Dorsal onlay • Urethral stricture

KEY POINTS

- Buccal mucosa is the preferred tissue for bulbar urethral stricture repair for strictures greater than 2 cm.
- Techniques for buccal mucosal placement include dorsal onlay, ventral onlay, lateral onlay, dorsal inlay, and a combined ventral onlay and dorsal inlay.
- Outcomes for the different graft locations are similar, approximately 90%.
- Location of the graft for bulbar stricture repair should be guided by surgeon experience and preference.

INTRODUCTION

The gold standard for bulbar urethroplasty has been excision and primary anastomosis (EPA), which involves excision of the strictured urethra and suturing of the healthy ends together. This method is durable and has a well-documented success rate of greater than 90%.[1,2] EPA is accepted as superior to less invasive approaches to treatment, such as urethral dilation and direct visualization and internal urethrotomy.[3] Application of this approach is generally limited to strictures that are 2 cm or less in the bulbar urethra due to potential penile shortening. Strictures greater than 2 cm are successfully treated with augmentation urethroplasty wherein the narrowed segment is not excised but widened with the use of a skin flap or, more commonly, a tissue graft.

Common modes of treatment of bulbar stricture include the following:

1. Urethral dilation
2. Direct visualization and internal urethrotomy
3. Urethroplasty
   a. EPA
   b. Augmented with tissue graft
      i. Dorsal onlay
      ii. Ventral onlay
      iii. Lateral onlay
      iv. Dorsal inlay
      v. Dorsal inlay, ventral onlay

GRAFTS: WHAT ARE THEY AND WHAT IS THEIR PURPOSE?

A graft is tissue that is isolated for the intended purpose of relocation and repair of a damaged recipient site. Once relocated, the site of interest must provide an environment amenable to acceptance of the transfer. A graft does not have an intrinsic blood supply and relies on a robust, nutrient-rich tissue bed for imbibition of nutrients during the first 48 hours, after which inosculation of new capillaries occurs.[4]

TYPES OF GRAFTS

There are 2 types of tissue grafts used in urethral reconstruction; they are differentiated by the amount of tissue transferred. A split-thickness

---

Conflicts of Interest: None.

Department of Urology, University of Minnesota, 420 Delaware Street South East, MMC 394, Minneapolis, MN 55455, USA

* Corresponding author.

E-mail address: selliott@umn.edu

http://dx.doi.org/10.1016/j.ucl.2016.08.009

urologic.theclinics.com

graft is limited to the epidermis and superficial dermal plexus. This plexus contains a plethora of small blood vessels making it favorable for graft–recipient site neovascularization. Conversely, the physical properties of this tissue are not well maintained; as a result, these grafts tend to contract and are less durable. Full-thickness skin grafts include the epidermis, the superficial dermal plexus, and the deep dermis. Given that the entire dermis is included, the tissue is relatively durable, with less propensity for contraction. Unlike the superficial dermal plexus, the deep dermis is sparsely populated with blood vessels making its acceptance of neovascularization from a donor bed potentially more challenging. One should avoid using hair-bearing skin for a full-thickness skin graft because the hair follicles are in the deep dermis and will result in inflammation, stone formation, and infection in the reconstructed urethra. This issue is not a concern with split-thickness grafts. An additional type of graft commonly used in reconstructive surgery is full-thickness mucosa. Mucosal tissue differs from skin in that it has the lamina propria as a subepidermal layer. This layer contains primarily connective tissue but also small blood vessels and lymphatics. The thinner this layer is, the easier neovascularization can transpire.[5–8]

HISTORY BEHIND GRAFT USE IN URETHRAL RECONSTRUCTION

There have been a myriad of different types of tissue used for the purpose of graft tissue transfer in urethral reconstructive surgery; some have been more successful than others. A favorable tissue type would include the following characteristics: easy to access and harvest, hairless, durable, viable in a wet environment, and a structure that facilitates neovascularization.[5–8]

Types of tissues attempted for urethroplasty grafts are as follows:

1. Split-thickness skin
2. Full-thickness skin
3. Bladder epithelium
4. Bowel mucosa
5. Oral mucosa

Split-thickness grafts have limited success when used for urethral stricture repair. This limited success is likely due to their higher rates of contracture, resulting in restricture, unsatisfactory cosmesis, diverticulum formation, postvoid dribbling, and ejaculatory dysfunction.[9,10] Full-thickness skin grafts from postauricular skin and the lateral abdominal wall have been described. Although no direct comparison exists and results are mixed, the full-thickness graft seems to be superior to the split-thickness graft. In comparison with mucosal grafts, some have reported higher rates of recurrence,[11] whereas other groups have reported similar rates.[12,13] The use of bladder epithelium was first described by Memmelaar[14] and in the modern era by Ransley and colleagues.[15] Colonic mucosal grafts have been described using both rectum and sigmoid mucosa.[16,17] Because of higher rates of recurrence and sacculation as well as a relatively invasive procurement, this type of tissue is not widely used.

Oral mucosa possesses many of the ideal graft characteristics for urethral reconstruction. From a technical standpoint, it is easily harvested with minimal morbidity. Additionally, its native environment is wet, similar to the urethra. Relative to bladder, rectum, and skin, it has a thick epithelium making it relatively durable and perhaps less prone to contracture or sacculation and has a thin lamina propria making it more receptive to expeditious neovasvularization.[5,6,8]

ORAL MUCOSAL GRAFTS

Target sites of oral mucosal graft include the cheek (buccal), lip (labial), and the tongue (lingual). Of these, buccal mucosa has the largest accessible surface area. Although it is involved in mastication and speaking, it is not as essential as the lip or tongue. Likely as a result, when compared with buccal grafts, labial and lingual have resulted in higher graft site morbidity.[18–20] In addition to favorable postoperative morbidity, the buccal graft contains the following features, making it an ideal candidate for graft tissue:

1. Easy to access and harvest
2. Hairless
3. Durable: full-thickness graft
4. Viable in a wet environment: native environment is the mouth
5. Structure that facilitates neovascularization: thin lamina propria

EVOLUTION OF THE USE OF ORAL MUCOSAL GRAFTS

Although many attribute British surgeon Graham Humby as the first to successfully use buccal mucosa for urethral reconstruction, it was initially described by the Russian urologist Kirill Sapezhko[21] in 1894.[22] Then in 1941, Humby[23] described a technique using buccal mucosa for hypospadias repair. The technique did not gain wide acceptance until the 1980s and 1990s. Although he did not use graft material, Monseur developed a technique in 1980 that laid the foundation for modern augmentation urethroplasty.[24] In Monseur's technique, he described a dorsal urethrotomy with the edges of the strictured urethra sutured to the underlying corporal bodies. Several groups began to publish their experience with buccal grafts in the early 1990s, including Burger and colleagues[25] in pediatric reconstruction and El-Kasaby and colleagues[26] and Duckett and colleagues[6] in adult reconstruction.

In bulbar stricture disease, techniques for different graft locations developed in the mid 1990s. In 1996, Barbagli and colleagues[27] modified the Monseur technique to include a dorsally placed buccal mucosal graft. During the same time, Morey and McAninch[28] described a ventral placement of the buccal graft. Subsequently, additional graft locations have been described, including lateral onlay,[29] dorsal inlay,[30] and a combination of dorsal inlay and ventral onlay.[31] Most surgical outcomes data are in the dorsal and ventral approaches to buccal placement. Most data involve retrospective single-site series making it challenging to establish definitive recommendations regarding the superiority of any one technique. The overwhelming data support similar outcomes of around 90%, regardless of graft location.[7,29,32,33] Therefore, the primary driving force behind technique selection should be surgeon preference. For the remainder of this review, the authors explore the following surgical techniques as well as clinic outcomes.

Oral mucosal graft placement locations are as follows:

1. Ventral onlay
2. Dorsal onlay
3. Dorsal inlay
4. Lateral onlay
5. Dorsal inlay and ventral onlay

DORSAL ONLAY BUCCAL MUCOSAL GRAFT
Surgical Technique

Barbagli and colleagues[27] initially described this surgical approach for bulbar stricture repair. Through a perineal incision, one divides the bulbospongiosus muscle and circumferentially isolates the bulbar urethra. A dorsal urethrotomy is made through the strictured urethra. The buccal graft is then sutured to the underlying tunica albuginea of the corpora cavernosa, both along the edges of the graft and across the face of the graft. This process, known as quilting, aids in the prevention of graft elevation from an underlying hematoma or seroma, potentially preventing graft neovascularization. Quilting may also prevent graft contraction.

The dorsally fixed buccal graft is then anastomosed to the urethrotomy site.

Although the graft itself is fixed to the dorsal urethra as well as corporal bodies, the surrounding muscles are completely freed, disrupting a portion of the native microvascular blood supply including circumflex and perforating arteries to the corpus spongiosum. Kulkarni and colleagues[34] modified Barbagli's approach by describing a unilateral urethral dissection with muscle preservation. The ischiocavernosus muscle is incised, allowing the urethra to be rotated dorsally with the bulbospongiosus muscle and the central tendon intact. The dissection is then further carried dorsally across the midline resulting in ample space for midline graft placement with only unilateral dissection. This technique is applicable to the more distal urethra as well, wherein the Buck fascia and its microvasculature can be left intact on one side (**Fig. 1**).

Advantages

1. Less blood loss
2. Intraoperative adaptability
3. More surrounding structural support

Given the eccentric shape of the bulbar urethra, most of the spongiosum is located ventrally.

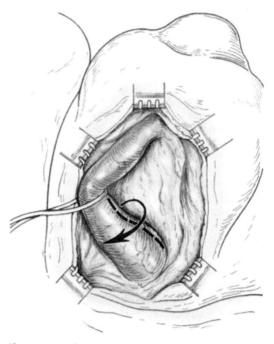

Fig. 1. Dorsal onlay approach to graft placement. *Dashed line* represents where the urethrotomy is made. (*From* Mangera A, Patterson JM, Chapple CR. A systematic review of graft augmentation urethroplasty techniques for the treatment of anterior urethral strictures. Eur Urol 2011;59:798; with permission.)

Thus, incision of the relatively thin dorsal spongiosum results in less continuous intraoperative blood loss. Although the blood loss during urethroplasty is never a danger to patients' health, it can impair visualization during exposure and graft placement, arguing in favor of dorsal placement. The dorsal approach to graft placement may also be preferred because it is the most versatile. Preoperative urethral imaging does not always corroborate with intraoperative findings, which may be a result of evolving stricture or suboptimal imaging. Therefore, the reconstructive surgeon must always have a plan B should one encounter pathology that was different or more extensive than initially anticipated. The dorsal approach has been successfully used in all locations of the urethra. The other graft locations, including ventral and lateral, have minimal application described in the literature outside of the bulbar urethra, thus, limiting their adaptability. If there is complete or near-complete obliteration of the urethra making a single augmentation graft impossible, one can enhance the dorsal graft with either an augmented anastomotic reconstruction[35] or a concurrent ventral onlay graft.[31] Additionally, the dorsal graft has more surrounding structural support given its fixation to the corporal bodies of the penis. This support potentially reduces sacculation and graft contraction. Sacculation may result in irritative voiding symptoms, urinary tract infections, postvoid dribbling, and impaired ejaculation.[35]

Disadvantages

1. Disruption of surrounding microvascular environment
2. Challenging visualization proximally
3. Dissection close to the membranous sphincter

Given the circumferential or unilateral dissection of the bulbar urethra, all or at a minimum some of the surrounding microvascular support is disrupted. This fact theoretically increases the possibility of graft failure. With review of the literature, there does not seem to be a significant difference in failure when compared with the minimal urethral dissection performed in ventral graft placement. Many are discouraged from performing proximal bulbar strictures that extend to the membranous urethra using a dorsal approach for concern about proximal visualization.[35] However, the authors have found that with careful dissection and stay sutures to facilitate rotation of the urethra, the proximal exposure can be equivalent to the ventral approach. Finally, in strictures that extend to the membranous urethra, the dorsal dissection is inside of the omega-shaped external urinary sphincter, which is more robust dorsally than

ventrally. This asymmetry is a concern for future continence, especially if the internal urinary sphincter is absent, as after a transurethral resection of the prostate. However, the authors and others have found that if the dissection stays very close to the spongiosum, a plane can be established between the sphincter and the urethra, thus, minimizing sphincter damage.

Outcomes

In 2011, Mangera and colleagues[36] published a meta-analysis regarding outcomes for urethroplasties involving graft placement. They identified 35 studies that looked at dorsal buccal graft outcomes. The mean success rate was 88.37%. Lower success rates were seen in series that included penile skin grafts. A subsequent meta-analysis in 2014 identified 66 studies and demonstrated an average success rate of 88.3% with an average follow-up of 42 months.[37]

VENTRAL ONLAY BUCCAL MUCOSAL GRAFT
Surgical Technique

Morey and McAninch[28] first described this surgical approach for bulbar stricture repair. A perineal incision is followed by a midline incision through the bulbospongiosus muscle. The muscle need not be reflected laterally from the corpus spongiosum, leaving the surrounding supportive structures intact. Once the stricture is located, a midline sagittal incision is made through the ventral spongiosum. The graft is then sewn directly to the edges of the urethrotomy. The outer adventitia of the corpus spongiosum is then closed over the graft, providing a vascular bed for neovascularization. A concern is that as this graft is free floating in the spongiosum, a hematoma may form between the graft and the spongiosum, impairing graft uptake. Furthermore, a lack of graft fixation may lead to sacculation. In response, the authors and others have modified the technique to include quilting sutures to the inner spongiosum before closing the outer adventitia layer. Like dorsal fixation, there are no data to support this additional step, but it follows sound surgical principles (**Fig. 2**).

Advantages

1. Minimal dissection
2. Robust blood supply in ventral sponge
3. Easier proximal exposure

As opposed to the dorsal approach, the ventral dissection is minimal, potentially resulting in reduced operative times. The minimal dissection of the bulbospongiosus muscles may also

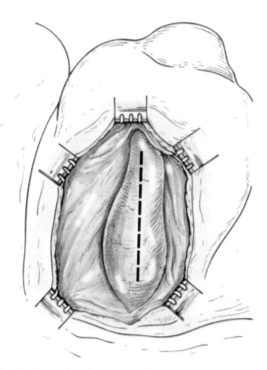

Fig. 2. Ventral onlay approach to graft placement. *Dashed line* represents where the urethrotomy is made. (*From* Mangera A, Patterson JM, Chapple CR. A systematic review of graft augmentation urethroplasty techniques for the treatment of anterior urethral strictures. Eur Urol 2011;59:798; with permission.)

minimize morbidity. Additionally the ventral portion of the bulbar urethra is significantly larger than the dorsal with a more robust direct blood supply than the tunica albuginea. Regarding exposure, there is no need for rotation of the urethra to gain access to the urethrotomy site. This more concise dissection allows for direct and potentially more straightforward proximal visualization and eventual graft placement.

Disadvantages

1. More blood loss
2. Less surrounding structural support
3. Less intraoperative adaptability

Conversely, because the ventral spongiosum is more robust, it also bleeds more vigorously. Although the need for blood transfusions is extremely rare, visualization is compromised by such blood flow, making graft placement challenging. Although again, the blood supply to the ventral sponge is rich, the tissue itself is not particularly firm compared with the strength of the underlying corporal bodies. Theoretically, there is an increased risk of graft sacculation, which could cause increased postvoid dribbling, urinary tract

infection, and ejaculatory dysfunction; these complications have not been widely reported in the literature.[35] Sacculation seems to be more evident in older series that used skin grafts.[38] Although rare, there is some documentation of urethrocutaneous fistula formation, not seen in the dorsally placed grafts.[39,40]

Outcomes

In Mangera and colleagues'[36] meta-analysis, they found 24 studies describing ventral graft outcomes with a mean surgical success of 88.84% and mean follow-up of 34.3 months. Subsequent reports have continued to demonstrate similar surgical success to dorsal placement.[41]

LATERAL ONLAY BUCCAL MUCOSAL GRAFT
Surgical Technique

The lateral graft placement, described by Barbagli and colleagues,[29] is an amalgam of the ventral and dorsal approaches. After one makes a midline sagittal incision in the bulbospongiosus muscle, one conducts a limited unilateral dissection, reflecting the muscle and freeing the corpus spongiosum from the underlying corporal bodies. Presumably this can be accomplished using the Kulkarni unilateral dissection technique described earlier. Of note, although the literature on this technique is sparse, this approach preceded the Kulkarni dorsal dissection. A lateral sagittal incision is made through the length of the stricture, and the graft is sewn in place in a similar fashion to the ventral approach (**Fig. 3**).

Advantages

1. Microvascular preservation
2. Enhanced visualized

Much like the Kulkarni unilateral dissection, this approach allows for preservation of the contralateral urethral blood supply. Given the eccentric orientation of the spongiosum, there may be less blood loss and improved visualization when performing the urethrotomy and graft placement.

Disadvantages

1. Less surrounding structural support
2. Less robust blood supply of recipient site

Given the lateral location of the graft, the corporal tissue support is absent from graft placement, similar to the ventral placement. There may be an increased propensity for sacculations in the graft. Additionally, the location carries less robust spongiosum blood supply than the ventral placement, similar to the dorsal approach but without the

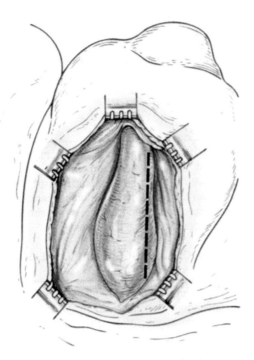

Fig. 3. Lateral onlay approach to graft placement. *Dashed line* represents where the urethrotomy is made. (*From* Mangera A, Patterson JM, Chapple CR. A systematic review of graft augmentation urethroplasty techniques for the treatment of anterior urethral strictures. Eur Urol 2011;59:798; with permission.)

underlying corporal bodies for graft support. This technique seems to incorporate the theoretic shortcomings of both the dorsal and ventral approaches without significant improvement in visualization or overall blood supply.

Outcomes

Data to support this approach are extremely limited. Barbagli and colleagues[29] reported a series of 6 patients with a 42-month follow-up. Outcomes were similar to dorsal and ventral populations within their study. There have been no subsequent articles on the approach; the limited uptake of this technique likely reflects its shortcomings compared with other approaches.

DORSAL INLAY BUCCAL MUCOSAL GRAFT
Surgical Technique

Asopa[30] developed a novel technique for dorsal placement of buccal mucosal grafts. Using an identical exposure to the ventral onlay approach, Asopa and colleagues[30] added to the procedure by following the ventral urethrotomy with a concurrent dorsal urethrotomy. Subsequently the split dorsal urethra is dissected free from the underlying corporal cavernosa. Once free bilaterally, the

dorsal urethral defect appears as an elliptical space of underlying tunica albuginea. The graft is quilted to the isolated tunica and secured laterally to the urethrotomy mucosal edges. The overlying ventral urethrotomy is closed in one or 2 layers per surgeon preference (**Fig. 4**).

Advantages

1. Minimal dissection
2. Preservation of native microvascular network
3. Easier proximal exposure
4. More surrounding structural support

The primary benefit of the dorsal inlay technique over the dorsal onlay is the ventral approach to stricture exposure and graft placement. The graft can be placed on the underlying support of the corpora cavernosa without the need for extensive urethral mobilization. This concise dissection theoretically preserves bilaterally the periurethral microvasculature as well as potentially preventing sacculation of the graft. Additionally there is relatively easier proximal exposure of the stricture compared with the dorsal approach.

Disadvantages

1. Reduced size of graft spread fixation relative to dorsal onlay

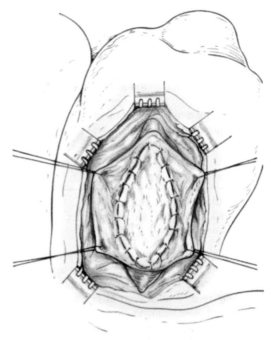

Fig. 4. Dorsal inlay approach to graft placement. (*From* Mangera A, Patterson JM, Chapple CR. A systematic review of graft augmentation urethroplasty techniques for the treatment of anterior urethral strictures. Eur Urol 2011;59:799; with permission.)

2. Greater than 1 urethrotomy
3. More blood loss

Compared with the dorsal onlay approach, the dorsal inlay graft contributes less to the increased urethral caliber. The limited mobilization results in a relatively smaller potential graft width, which may limit the applicability of this approach in narrow strictures. Additionally, there is more than one urethrotomy, potentially increasing the possibility of blood loss, urethral stricture, or fistula formation, although none of these complications has been documented in the literature.[33,42,43] Furthermore, in very narrow strictures, the double urethrotomy leaves very little urethral epithelium on the 2 lateral strips to sew to both the graft and the ventral midline urethral closure.

Outcomes

Asopa and colleagues[30] reported surgical success at a rate of 87%. Several other reports subsequently have found success rates equivalent to the dorsal onlay approach, ranging from 87% to 92%.[33,42,43] Aldaqadossi and colleagues[33] conducted a prospective randomized study of individuals having either dorsal onlay or dorsal inlay graft placement. They found a significant decrease in operative times and blood loss with the dorsal inlay group.

DORSAL INLAY AND VENTRAL ONLAY BUCCAL MUCOSAL GRAFT
Surgical Technique

In 2007, Palminteri and colleagues[44] described a technique for stricture repair using both ventrally and dorsally placed small intestinal submucosal grafts and, later, a series using buccal mucosa.[31] The approach involves a similar dissection to the dorsal inlay technique with an additional ventrally placed buccal mucosal graft. Thus, there are double overlapping buccal grafts both ventrally and dorsally.

Advantages

1. Largest potential increase in caliber of urethra
2. Minimal dissection
3. Preservation of native microvascular network
4. Easier proximal exposure

This technique was largely developed for the pinpoint urethral stricture for which a single graft would be insufficient for a normal-caliber urethra. The dorsal inlay does not provide the same caliber potential as the dorsal onlay; with the addition of the ventral onlay, maximal diameter can be achieved. Much like the ventral onlay

and dorsal inlay techniques, minimal periurethral dissection is required resulting in an increase in the preserved native surrounding vasculature and a possible reduction in operative time. Furthermore, easier proximal exposure of the urethral stricture is achieved because of the ventral approach (**Fig. 5**).

Disadvantages

1. Less surrounding structural support of ventral graft
2. Increased demand of graft material
3. Greater than 1 urethrotomy
4. More blood loss

Much like the isolated ventral onlay, the dorsal inlay/ventral onlay technique has the potential for increased sacculation and resulting postvoid and postejaculation dribbling. Given that both ventral and dorsal grafts are placed, there is an increased demand of graft material. Patient factors may limit graft supply, making this approach more challenging. Additionally, like with the dorsal inlay technique, there is more than one urethrotomy. Increased incisions theoretically could result in a higher stricture or fistula rate and increased potential intraoperative blood loss, but these complications have not been documented in the literature.[31,44,45]

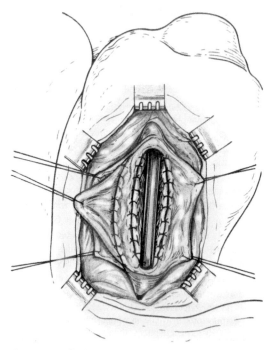

Fig. 5. Dorsal inlay and ventral onlay approach to graft placement. (*From* Mangera A, Patterson JM, Chapple CR. A systematic review of graft augmentation urethroplasty techniques for the treatment of anterior urethral strictures. Eur Urol 2011;59:799; with permission.)

Outcomes

With small intestinal submucosal graft used for dorsal inlay/ventral onlay, Palminteri and colleagues[31] found 85% success with an average follow-up of 21 months.[44] With buccal mucosa, Palminteri and colleagues[31] found 89.6% success at an average of 22 months of follow-up. At an average of 49 months, they found consistent surgical success and no associated sexual dysfunction.[45]

SUMMARY

In experienced hands, the success of oral mucosal graft for urethroplasty is similar regardless of location. Although there are subtle theoretic benefits to each graft location, data have not supported a significant long-term difference in success. First and foremost, surgeons should select a technique with which they feel comfortable. If there is a high likelihood of extension beyond the bulbar urethra, one should consider dorsal placement of the graft given the versatility of this approach. Should there be complete or almost-complete obliteration of the urethra, one may consider a double overlapping buccal mucosal graft. Regardless of approach, surgeon experience as well as appropriate patient expectations of procedural success will lead to optimal surgical results.

REFERENCES

1. Santucci RA, Mario LA, McAninch JW. Anastomotic urethroplasty for bulbar urethral stricture: analysis of 168 patients. J Urol 2002;167:1715–9.
2. Barbagli G, Guazzoni G, Lazzeri M. One-stage bulbar urethroplasty: retrospective analysis of the results in 375 patients. Eur Urol 2008;53:828–33.
3. Santucci R, Eisenberg L. Urethrotomy has a much lower success rate than previously reported. J Urol 2010;183:1859–62.
4. Jordan GH. The application of tissue transfer techniques in urologic surgery. In: Webster G, Kirby R, King L, et al, editors. Reconstructive urology. Oxford (United Kingdom): Blackwell Scientific; 1993. p. 143–69.
5. Baskin LS, Duckett JW. Mucosal grafts in hypospadias and stricture management. AUA Update Series 1994;XIII:270.
6. Duckett JW, Coplen D, Ewalt D, et al. Buccal mucosal urethral replacement. J Urol 1995;153(5): 1660–3.
7. Venkatesan K, Blakely S, Nikolavsky D. Surgical repair of bulbar urethral strictures: advantages of ventral, dorsal, and lateral approaches and when to choose them. Adv Urol 2015;2015:397936.
8. Zimmerman WB, Santucci RA. Buccal mucosa urethroplasty for adult urethral strictures. Indian J Urol 2011;27:364–70.
9. Blum JA, Feeney MJ, Howe GE, et al. Skin patch urethroplasty: 5 year follow-up. J Urol 1982; 127(5):909.
10. Wessells H, McAninch JW. Use of free grafts in urethral stricture reconstruction. J Urol 1996;155: 1912–5.
11. Liu JS, Han J, Said M, et al. Long-term outcomes of urethroplasty with abdominal wall skin grafts. Urology 2015;85(1):258–62.
12. Hudak SJ, Hudson TC, Morey AF. 'Minipatch' penile skin graft urethroplasty in the era of buccal mucosal grafting. Arab J Urol 2012;10(4):378–81.
13. Palminteri E, Berdondini E, Lumen N, et al. Kulkarni dorsolateral graft urethroplasty using penile skin. Urology 2016;90:179–83.
14. Memmelaar J. Use of bladder mucosa in a one-stage repair of hypospadias. J Urol 1947;58:68–73.
15. Ransley PG, Duffy PG, Van Oesch IL, et al. The use of bladder mucosa and combined bladder mucosa/preputial skin grafts for urethral reconstruction. J Urol 1987;138:1096–8.
16. Palmer DA, Marcello PW, Zinman LN, et al. Urethral reconstruction with rectal mucosa graft onlay: a novel minimally invasive technique. J Urol 2016; 196:782–6.
17. Xu YM, Qiao Y, Sa YL, et al. Urethral reconstruction using colonic mucosa graft for complex strictures. J Urol 2009;182(3):1040–3.
18. Sharma AK, Chandrashekar R, Keshavamurthy R, et al. Lingual versus buccal mucosa graft urethroplasty for anterior urethral stricture: a prospective comparative analysis. Int J Urol 2013;20(12): 1199–203.
19. Kamp S, Knoll T, Osman M, et al. Donor-site morbidity in buccal mucosa urethroplasty: lower lip or inner cheek? BJU Int 2005;96(4):619–23.
20. Lumen N, Vierstraete-Verlinde S, Oosterlinck W, et al. Buccal versus lingual mucosa graft in anterior urethroplasty: a prospective comparison of surgical outcome and donor site morbidity. J Urol 2016; 195(1):112–7.
21. Sapezhko KM. On treatments of urethral defects by the way of mucosal transplantation. Khirurgicheskaya Letopis 1894;4:775–83.
22. Korneyev I, Ilyin D, Schulthesiss D, et al. The first oral mucosal graft urethroplasty was carried out in the 19th century: the pioneering experience of Kirill Sapezhko (1857-1928). Eur Urol 2012;62(4): 624–7.
23. Humby GA. One-stage operation for hypospadias repair. Br J Surg 1941;29:84–92.
24. Monseur J. Widening of the urethra using the supra-urethral layer (author's transl) [in French]. J Urol 1980;86:439–49.

25. Burger RA, Muller SC, El-Damanhoury H, et al. The buccal mucosal graft for urethral reconstruction: a preliminary report. J Urol 1992;147(3):662–4.

26. El-Kasaby AW, Fath-Alla M, Noweir AM. The use of buccal mucosa patch graft in the management of anterior urethral strictures. J Urol 1993;149(2): 276–8.

27. Barbagli G, Selli C, Tosto A, et al. Dorsal free graft urethroplasty. J Urol 1996;155(1):123–6.

28. Morey AF, McAninch JW. Technique of harvesting buccal mucosa for urethral reconstruction. J Urol 1996;155(5):1696–7.

29. Barbagli G, Palminteri E, Guazzoni G, et al. Bulbar urethroplasty using buccal mucosa grafts placed on the ventral, dorsal, or lateral surface of the urethra: are results affected by the surgical technique? J Urol 2005;174:955–7.

30. Asopa HS, Garg M, Singhal GG, et al. Dorsal free graft urethroplasty for urethral stricture by ventral sagittal urethrotomy approach. Urol 2001;58:657–9.

31. Palminteri E, Manzoni G, Berdondini E, et al. Combined dorsal plus ventral double buccal mucosa graft in bulbar urethral reconstruction. Eur Urol 2008;53:81–9.

32. Wang K, Miao X, Wang L, et al. Dorsal onlay versus ventral onlay urethroplasty for anterior urethral stricture: a meta-analysis. Urol Int 2009;83:342–8.

33. Aldaqadossi H, El Gamal S, El-Nadey M, et al. Dorsal onlay (Barbagli technique) versus dorsal inlay (Asopa technique) buccal mucosal graft urethroplasty for anterior urethral stricture: a prospective randomized study. Int J Urol 2014;21:185–8.

34. Kulkarni S, Barbagli G, Sansalone S, et al. One sided anterior urethroplasty: a new dorsal onlay graft technique. BJU Int 2009;104(8):1150–5.

35. Patterson JM, Chapple CR. Surgical techniques in substitution urethroplasty using buccal mucosa for the treatment of anterior urethral strictures. Eur Urol 2008;53(6):1162–71.

36. Mangera A, Patterson JM, Chapple CR. A systematic review of graft augmentation urethroplasty techniques for the treatment of anterior urethral strictures. Eur Urol 2011;59:797–814.

37. Chapple C, Andrich D, Atala A, et al. SIU/ICUD consultation on urethral strictures: the management of anterior urethral stricture disease using substitution urethroplasty. Urology 2014;83(3 Suppl):S31–47.

38. Bhargava S, Chapple CR. Buccal mucosal urethroplasty: is it the new gold standard? BJU Int 2004; 93(9):1191–3.

39. Andrich DE, Leach CJ, Mundy AR. The Barbagli procedure gives the best results for patch urethroplasty of the bulbar urethra. BJU Int 2001;88(4):385–9.

40. Fichtner J, Filipas D, Fisch M, et al. Long-term outcomes of ventral buccal mucosa onlay graft urethroplasty for urethral stricture repair. Urology 2004; 64(4):648–50.

41. Vasudeva P, Nanda B, Kumar A, et al. Dorsal versus ventral onlay buccal mucosal graft urethroplasty for long-segment bulbar urethral stricture: a prospective randomized study. Int J Urol 2015;22(10): 967–71.

42. Gupta NP, Ansari MS, Dogra PN, et al. Dorsal buccal mucosal graft urethroplasty by a ventral sagittal urethrotomy and minimal-access perineal approach for anterior urethral stricture. BJU Int 2004;93:1287–90.

43. Pisapati VL, Paturi S, Bethu S, et al. Dorsal buccal mucosal graft urethroplasty for anterior urethral stricture by Asopa technique. Eur Urol 2009;56:201–5.

44. Palminteri E, Berdondini E, Colombo F, et al. Small intestinal submucosal (SIS) graft urethroplasty: short term-term results. Eur Urol 2007;51:1695–701.

45. Palminteri E, Berdondini E, Shokeir AA, et al. Two-sided bulbar urethroplasty using dorsal plus ventral oral graft: urinary and sexual outcomes of a new technique. J Urol 2011;185:1766–71.

Sexual Dysfunction After Urethroplasty

Prem Nath Dogra, MCh, DSc (Hon)*, Prabhjot Singh, MCh, Rishi Nayyar, MCh, Siddharth Yadav, MS

KEYWORDS

- Sexual dysfunction • Urethroplasty • Erectile dysfunction • Urethral stricture • Sexuality preserving

KEY POINTS

- With the voiding function taken care of, the focus is shifting towards the inadvertent complications of urethroplasty, such as sexual dysfunction (SD).
- De novo posturethroplasty SD is uncommon—approximately 1% (0%–38%) after anterior urethroplasty and approximately 3% (0%–34%) after pelvic fracture urethral injury (PFUI) repair.
- The time of assessment and the type of urethroplasty may affect sexual outcomes.
- For bulbar strictures, nontransecting procedures may provide better sexual outcomes compared with excision and anatomosis.
- Although posterior urethroplasty has the highest chance of SD, most of it is attributable to the fracture itself rather than the urethroplasty.

INTRODUCTION

Urethroplasty is considered the standard of care for urethral stricture disease. With its superior long-term success rates, little morbidity, and cost-effectiveness, it has largely replaced endoscopic procedures as the current gold standard.[1,2] The goal of urethroplasty is to restore voiding function; thus, most of the available literature uses this criterion to define success. With good long-term success rates of urethroplasty addressing voiding function, focus is shifting toward inadvertent complications, such as SD.[3–5] As with any other genital surgery, there is a possibility of injury to the cavernous nerves or to the pudendal artery or a chance of penile shortening, which can affect postoperative sexual function. It was Mundy,[6] in 1993, who first reported permanent erectile dysfunction after urethroplasty. In their study of 200 patients, the rate of permanent erectile dysfunction after anastomotic transperineal and abdominoperineal urethroplasty was 5% and that after graft urethroplasty was 0.9%. Corsey and colleagues[7] in 2001 echoed Mundy's results and showed that the overall satisfaction with erection worsened in 30.9% of the patients after urethroplasty, but also noted a worsening of erection in 27.3% of patients in the control group who underwent circumcision. These contradictory findings sparked a debate and led to further evaluation among reconstructive urologists. Currently, there is a growing concern about the ill effects of urethroplasty on the various aspects of sexual function and certain ways have been proposed to reduce or prevent it.

EVALUATION AND QUESTIONNAIRES

Normal sexual function is a result of complex interplay between vascular, nervous, endocrinologic, and psychological systems leading to erection,

Financial Disclosures: None for all authors.
Conflicts of Interest: None for all authors.
Department of Urology, All India Institute of Medical Sciences, Room 5030, 5th Floor, Teaching Block, New Delhi 110029, India
* Corresponding author.
E-mail address: premnathdogra@gmail.com

Urol Clin N Am 44 (2017) 49–56
http://dx.doi.org/10.1016/j.ucl.2016.08.013

ejaculation, orgasm, and overall satisfaction. From a patient's standpoint, baseline sexual function, cause of the stricture, psychological impact of the stricture or its treatment, postoperative tissue edema or inflammation, or the urethroplasty itself may lead to posturethroplasty SD.[8] Sexual function can be assessed using standard validated questionnaires, such as the International Index of Erectile Function, International Index of Erectile Function – 5, Sexual Health Inventory for Men, O'Leary Brief Male Sexual Function Inventory, and Male Sexual Health Questionnaire for Ejaculatory Dysfunction, but none of these is specific to the posturethroplasty setting. The only validated questionnaire for urethroplasty does not assess changes in the sexual function.[9] Thus, various nonvalidated in-house questionnaires are being used and reported, making comparison among different studies difficult. One such questionnaire, the Post-Urethroplasty Sexual Questionnaire, specifically assesses changes in sexual function after urethroplasty and includes domains, such as genital sensitivity, genital cosmesis, satisfaction after urethroplasty, and the importance of counseling.[5] Another posturethroplasty questionnaire combines the Sexual Health Inventory for Men and Male Sexual Health Questionnaire for Ejaculatory Dysfunction with urethroplasty-specific questions, such as the effect of surgery on the sexual function, postoperative alteration in the penile length, and curvature and genital sensitivity, including glans tumescence and cold feeling of the glans.[10] Various other in-house nonvalidated questionnaires have been used for this purpose but a standard validated uniform questionnaire to assess the sexual outcomes after urethroplasty is still lacking.[11] This review discusses de novo SD after urethroplasty (anterior and posterior urethra), its proposed mechanisms, and the proposed ways to prevent or reduce it.

DE NOVO SEXUAL DYSFUNCTION: EFFECT OF URETHROPLASTY ON VARIOUS ASPECTS OF SEXUAL FUNCTION

SD is a broad term and for a posturethroplasty patient it encompasses erectile dysfunction, ejaculatory dysfunction, penile curvature or chordee, and genital sensitivity disorders. Current available literature suggests that the de novo posturethroplasty SD is uncommon, approximately 1% (0%–38%) after anterior urethroplasty and approximately 3% (0%–34%) after PFUI repair.[12,13] Postoperative de novo erectile dysfunction can result from an injury to the bulbar artery or to the vascular connections between the cavernosa and the spongiosa during the mobilization of the bulbar

urethra or from an injury to the cavernous nerves during the intercrural dissection of the urethra (cavernous nerves run at 1 o'clock and 11 o'clock positions, 3 mm outside the spongiosa).[5,12,14,15] The ejaculatory function can either improve or deteriorate after urethroplasty. Relief of the urethral obstruction leads to an increase in the force of ejaculation and reduces the associated burning or pain, thus improving postoperative ejaculation.[5] Whereas injury to the bulbospongiosus muscle (division and retraction of muscle to expose the bulbar urethra) or to the perineal nerves (perineal nerves may be injured during the dissection of central tendon as they emerge from ischiorectal fossa or small branches of the perineal nerve may be injured while dividing and retracting the bulbospongiosus muscle) may lead to reduced stream of ejaculation or postejaculatory dribbling. Weakening of a ventrally placed graft (pseudodiverticula formation) may also result in ejaculatory dysfunction.[5,16] Shortening of the urethra after excision and anastomosis for a long bulbar urethral stricture may result in a new-onset penile curvature and chordee. The mobilization and transection of spongiosa required for primary anastomosis may lead to poor blood flow distal to the transection, resulting in postoperative cold glans and poor glans tumescence during erections.[5,17] Injury to the perineal nerves, which provide sensory supply to perineum, scrotum, and the ventral surface of the shaft of penis, may result in postoperative genital sensitivity disorders.[16] Lastly, the psychological stress of the stricture disease and the recent surgery and postsurgery tissue inflammation and edema may also contribute to the SD.[8] Therefore, urethroplasty can affect multiple domains of sexual function and postsurgery SD is multifactorial in origin.

FACTORS AFFECTING POSTURETHROPLASTY SEXUAL FUNCTION

A patient's age, length of stricture, previous interventions, and type of urethroplasty have been proposed to affect posturethroplasty sexual function, but evidence is mostly lacking. Posturethroplasty erectile dysfunction was initially shown to be higher in older patients with longer strictures (6.8 cm vs 4.4 cm).[7] Further studies have refuted this association, however, and a recent meta-analysis found no association between the length of the stricture and the incidence of postoperative erectile dysfunction.[12,14] Similarly, Erickson and colleagues[18] showed that patients greater than 50 years old had a higher decline in erectile function after urethroplasty, but these findings were not reproduced by others and the association between age, length of stricture, previous surgeries, and posturethroplasty SD is unclear.

Sexual function in the immediate postoperative period is poor and as the healing occurs, it tends to improve. Dogra and colleagues,[14] in their prospective analysis of patients undergoing anterior urethroplasty, showed that the erectile function is worst at 3 months after surgery and then recovers to the preoperative level in most patients at approximately 6 months and then remains stable. Similarly, another study showed the postoperative erectile function to be significantly better in patients more than 1 year after urethroplasty compared with those within the first year.[4] This transient decline in the erectile function has been attributed to dissection or thermal injury (electrocautery)–induced neuropraxia of the cavernous nerves or to the postoperative hematoma and inflammation at the surgical site along with the psychological effects of the surgery.[17] A similar recovery in the ejaculatory function after bulbar anastomotic urethroplasty was noted by Beysens and colleagues[17] at 6 months of follow-up. Thus, the timing of assessment is important. At 6 months to 1-year postsurgery, the sexual function returns to the baseline level with no residual effect in most of the patients. There is a residual permanent de novo erectile dysfunction in a small percentage, however, which is the cause of dissatisfaction even after a successful surgery. Available literature, almost unanimously, shows no difference in the posturethoplasty SD rates between the different locations of the stricture or the type of the urethroplasty performed.[12] There is some evidence, however, that posterior urethroplasty carries the highest risk of erectile dysfunction, and in anterior urethroplasties, especially for short bulbar strictures, the nontransecting procedures may better preserve sexual function compared with transecting procedures but the debate continues.[5,17]

SEXUAL DYSFUNCTION AFTER ANTERIOR URETHROPLASTY

Bulbar urethroplasty poses greater risk of injury to cavernosal nerves and the vascular supply, thus has higher chances of postoperative SD.[4,5,19] Problems, such as impaired erection and ejaculation, are more frequent after bulbar urethroplasty, whereas, penile curvature and cosmesis are the primary concerns after penile urethroplasty (**Table 1**).[4]

Penile Urethroplasty

Penile urethral strictures are usually managed by dorsal graft urethroplasty and penile flaps are currently seldom used. If the stricture is long, tight, complex, or associated with lichen sclerosis or there is a history of previously failed repair, the procedure can be staged. Various investigators have assessed the impact of different types of urethroplasty on sexual function and mostly no significant differences could be established. Most of these studies were limited, however, by small sample size, heterogeneous patient group, and varied timing of assessment. Penile flap procedures can lead to a decline in the erectile function in approximately 40% and a major change in erectile length and angle in 20% of the cases, which results in a decline in intercourse frequency, leading to overall dissatisfaction in 27% of the patients.[7] Although statistically insignificant, penile flap procedures affect the sexual functions the most.[7] Over the years, the surgery for long penile strictures has moved away from flap procedures to grafting. The impact of graft penile urethroplasty on sexual function is more favorable and is almost

Table 1
Reported rates of sexual dysfunction after different types of urethroplasties

Type of Urethroplasty	Erectile Dysfunction (%)	Ejaculatory Dysfunction (%)	Chordee/ Curvature (%)	Reduced Glans Turgidity or Coldness	Genital Sensitivity
Anterior urethroplasty					
Penile flap	40[7]	NA	27.3[7]	NA	NA
Penile graft	4.5–19.2[7,10,14]	20[4]	15.4–23[7,10]	NA	45[10]
Bulbar transecting	1–50[4,7,11,14,23,24,49]	10.8–23.3[11,23]	5–26.6[7,24,26]	10–16.7[7,17,26]	18.3–58[11,23,26]
Bulbar nontransecting	1–26[4,14,26,28]	0–19[5,26,28]	0[5,27,28]	4–60[5,17,26]	40–42[5,26]
Posterior urethroplasty					
Overall	25–86[13,37,38]	NA	NA	NA	NA
De novo	2–5[8,13,]	3–8.6[34,49]	NA	NA	NA

similar to that of bulbar urethroplasty (postoperative dysfunction rates 16%–25%).[4,12,14] There is no relation between the length of the penile stricture or the graft and the incidence of postoperative erectile dysfunction. Erickson and colleagues[4] assessed ejaculatory function after penile graft urethroplasty and found a stable function in most of the patients. Staging the procedure of graft urethroplasty for pananterior urethral strictures does not seem to adversely affect the sexual functions and the outcomes are similar to that of a single-stage procedure.[10] Xie and colleagues[20] assessed erectile dysfunction after graft urethroplasty for complex pananterior urethral strictures (>10 cm long, either single or at multiple sites) and observed transient penile edema in 5 patients, penile shortening in 6 patients, and an erectile dysfunction rate of 25% at 6 months postsurgery. They suggested an overall low rate of SD as long the stricture did not extend into proximal bulbar urethra or required intercrural dissection. Thus, graft urethroplasty limited to penile urethra leads to temporary erectile dysfunction in patients 20% of the patients, which recovers in most at 6 months after surgery.

Bulbar Urethroplasty

Bulbar urethral strictures are managed either by transecting techniques (ie, excision and primary or augmented anastomosis) or by nontransecting techniques (ie, graft urethroplasty).[1] The management of a short obliterative or a long-segment bulbar stricture is straightforward: excision and anastomosis as the only options for an obliterative stricture and grafting for the long segment stricture. It is the short-segment nonobliterative bulbar stricture, in which both excision and grafting are suitable, that is the cause of debate. Transection is preferred for traumatic strictures, which usually have an obliterative transmural spongiofibrosis, and nontransecting technique is usually reserved for idiopathic strictures, where the spongiofibrosis is superficial and can be excised without the need of transection.

Transecting techniques
Short-segment uncomplicated or obliterative bulbar strictures are amenable to complete excision with primary anastomosis, which is considered as the most successful treatment.[11,21,22] Several studies have assessed sexual outcomes after excision and end to end anastomosis and noted a new-onset erectile dysfunction in 21.4% and an ejaculatory dysfunction in 20% of the patients and in 3.3% ejaculation was only possible by manual compression of perineum at the level of the urethral bulb. Neurovascular disorders,

such as cold glans, poor glans tumescence, and sensitivity, were noted in 31.6% and new-onset penile curvature was noted in 3.6% of the cases. Despite that all these patients were recurrence-free at 5 years postsurgery, 2 (3%) patients were still dissatisfied by the surgery.[11,23] Similar poor sexual outcomes have been reported after excision and primary anastomosis for a long (>2.5 cm) bulbar stricture along with a higher chance of postoperative chordee.[24] Therefore, the authors suggested that longer bulbar strictures are better managed by excision followed by augmented roof strip anastomosis, which has similar SD profile with no increased risk of chordee.[23] Thus, despite its excellent success rates, there is a high chance of SD after transecting bulbar urethroplasty resulting from the damage to the bulbospongiosus muscle or the perineal nerve, the transection of spongiosal blood supply, or the shortening of urethra resulting in erectile, ejaculatory, and other types of SD.[5,11]

Nontransecting techniques
The longer bulbar urethral strictures (>2–3 cm) are mostly managed by nontransecting graft urethroplasty. Keeping the corpora spongiosa intact preserves the blood supply to the glans, theoretically giving the same benefits as the bulbar artery–sparing techniques.[24] Palminteri and colleagues[5] assessed the impact of ventral onlay graft urethroplasty on postoperative sexual functions and observed a worsened ejaculation in 19% and cold glans in only 4% of the patients with preserved erectile function in all at 1 year of follow-up. Worsened ejaculatory function was attributed to the weakening of the ventrally placed graft with pseudodiverticula formation and the investigators concluded that a nontransecting ventral urethroplasty may protect against postoperative SD.

Transecting versus nontransecting bulbar urethroplasty
Several investigators have evaluated whether the nontransecting is superior to the transecting bulbar urethroplasty in terms of sexual outcomes. The rates of erectile dysfunction, ejaculatory dysfunction, and impaired glans turgidity were similar between the 2 groups, with a slightly higher chance of penile angulation or shortening after excision and anastomosis.[17,25] But the success rate of urethroplasty was higher in excision group compared with grafting and the current evidence suggests that the 2 procedures have almost similar effects on the sexual functions and the difference, if any, is small.

Other techniques and modifications

Injury to the bulbar artery during the dissection and transection of corpus spongiosum is one of the causes of the posturethroplasty SD.[5,11] For a short-segment proximal bulbar urethral stricture, Jordan and colleagues[26] described a technique of bulbar artery–sparing end-to-end anastomosis, which would theoretically avoid reduced glans turgidity and sensitivity even after spongiosal transection. Posturethroplasty ejaculatory dysfunction is attributed to the weakening of a ventrally placed graft or to the damage to the bulbospongiosus muscle or to the perineal nerves. Palminteri and colleagues[5] suggested ways to reduce risk of postoperative ejaculatory disorders by careful midline opening of the bulbospongiosus, no sectioning of the central perineal tendon, covering the graft with spongiosa, and reconstructing the bulbospongiosus muscle. Even if the muscle is split carefully in midline, the muscle fibers and the perineal nerve fibers running laterally over the muscle may be damaged by retraction and thus even after reapproximation it may not function.[16] To overcome this, Barbagali and colleagues[16] described a modified technique for graft bulbar urethroplasty suitable for both ventral and dorsal graft placement that avoids division of the bulbospongiosus muscle or central perineal tendon. None of the 12 patients who underwent nerve and muscle–sparing graft bulbar urethroplasty (6 ventral and 6 dorsal onlay) reported a decrease in the force of ejaculation or postvoid dribbling or pseudodiverticulae formation at 12 months of follow-up.

Due to the higher chance of SD associated with excision and primary repair, some investigators prefer graft urethroplasty. But for a tight stricture (unable to pass 7F rigid ureteroscope or <3 mm diameter), placement of a graft may not result in an adequate urethral lumen and forces excision and anastomosis. Palminteri and colleagues[27,28] proposed a novel urethra-sparing technique for tight bulbar urethral strictures using a combination of dorsal and ventral grafts, augmenting the urethra on both sides and achieving an adequate lumen. This double-graft technique preserves the urethral plate and avoids sexual complications and chordee.[28] Of the 12 patients assessed, none reported postoperative erectile dysfunction, penile curvature, or shortening. Despite its excellent sexual outcomes, the reported long-term success rate of this procedure is 89.6%, which is lower than that reported for excision and primary anastomosis.

Although the position of graft placement has never been compared in terms of sexual outcomes, it is proposed that placing the graft dorsally might impair erection by risking injury to the cavernosal nerves and the bulbar arteries, especially when the dissection is very proximal, leading to possible postoperative erectile dysfunction. On the other hand, ventral grafting is technically easier, requires less urethral dissection and mobilization, and can be considered sexually safe. But there is a higher chance of pseudodiverticula formation with subsequent poor postoperative ejaculation and postejaculatory dribble.[28]

In some cases, the stricture may extend into the membranous urethra and because of fear of incontinence and impotence such strictures are usually managed endoscopically.[29] Blakely and colleagues[30] reported on sexual outcomes in 16 men who underwent dorsal onlay buccal mucosal graft urethroplasty for transurethral resection of prostate or radiation-induced long strictures involving membranous and bulbomembranous urethra and noted new-onset mild erectile dysfunction in only 1 patient. The investigators concluded that by avoiding circumferential dissection and transection of the urethra, there was a little effect on erectile function despite the resection of fibrotic tissue in the intercrural space.

POSTERIOR URETHROPLASTY

Pelvic fractures result from high-velocity injuries and are associated with genitourinary tract injury in 11% to 30% of the cases and urethral injury in approximately 10%.[30–32] Pelvic fracture itself is associated with a high incidence of erectile dysfunction, which can be attributed to neurogenic, vasculogenic, corporal, or psychogenic causes. Using penile duplex ultrasonography, arteriogram, and response to intracavernosal injections, Schenfeld and colleagues[33] reported that most of the cases of erectile dysfunction are of neurogenic etiology (72%) compared with vasculogenic etiology (28%). Cavernosal nerves and pudendal artery branches, which run near the apex of the prostate and pass under the pubic bones through urogenital diaphragm, are often injured in pelvic fracture.[13] Direct injury to the corporal bodies leading to intracorporal fibrosis or venous leakage or the associated psychological stress may also contribute to the postinjury poor erectile function.[30] High severity of trauma, tiles type B or C pelvic fractures, bilateral pubic rami fractures, marked pubic diastasis, and the associated urethral injury increase the chances of postinjury erectile dysfunction.[30,34] SD is noted in 35.9% (14%–72%) of men and 39.6% (31%–66.6%) of women after pelvic fracture and those who recover do so by 18 months' postinjury.[32,35,36]

Early studies reported a high incidence of erectile dysfunction after urethroplasty for PFUIs, with severe erectile dysfunction rates as high as 30%, but most of these are attributable to pelvic fracture itself rather than the urethroplasty (see **Table 1**).[34] In a large retrospective analysis of 573 patients who underwent anastomotic urethroplasty for PFUI, no difference was noted between the rates of preurethroplasty (posttrauma) (85%) and posturethroplasty (86%) erectile dysfunction.[37] Even in patients with complex posterior urethral disruptions (>3-cm gap, associated perineal or rectourethral fistulas, false passages, or an open bladder neck), no change in potency status was noted after combined abdominal transpubic perineal urethroplasty.[38] These studies support the suggestion that the urethral injury is a surrogate marker for severity of pelvic injury, and the pelvic injury itself rather than the urethroplasty is the cause of erectile dysfunction. El-Assmy and colleagues[39] and Anger and colleagues[40] recorded the ejaculatory function after repair of PFUI and reported good postoperative ejaculatory function, with only a few patients complaining of decreased force and volume (17.2%), delayed (8.6%) or dry ejaculations (1.7%). Post-PFUI erectile dysfunction may even improve after urethroplasty, with 16% to 66% of the patients who were impotent after injury regaining their erectile function postsurgery.[41,42] Thus, there are a few deleterious effects of posterior urethroplasty on sexual function, which may even improve with excision of fibrous scar tissue impinging on the cavernosal nerves or because of psychological effects of the successful treatment.

TREATMENT

Treatment of posturethroplasty erectile dysfunction is similar to that of other causes of erectile dysfunction. PDE5Is, which are the current first-line treatment of erectile dysfunction, have been tried in posturethroplasty setting. Most patients with post-anterior urethroplasty erectile dysfunction respond to PDE5Is, whereas for PFUI, treatment success depends on the etiology of erectile dysfunction, with a 60% improvement for neurogenic causes and 20% for arteriogenic causes, and an overall response rate of 47% to 80%.[32,43] If they fail, intracavernosal injection can be used with a 100% success rate in neurogenic causes and an approximately 50% success rate in arteriogenic causes of erectile dysfunction.[32]

Surgical management with penile revascularization can be offered to selected patients with PFUI with arteriogenic cause of erectile dysfunction who have failed more conservative management. Surgical repair is advocated for less than 55-year-old, nondiabetic nonsmokers with an isolated occlusion of the internal pudendal artery and no venous leak.[44] Success rate of such a procedure using inferior epigastric artery in this setting is approximately 50%.[45] Penile prosthesis is the last resort for patients who have failed medical treatment with a 90% to 100% chance of patient and partner satisfaction.[46]

PDE5Is are also used in penile rehabilitation after PFUI as a single daily dose for 3 months with good overall response rates. Those who present for treatment within 1 month of injury and have some nocturnal erections have better outcomes compared with those presenting late or have no nocturnal erections.[47,48]

SUMMARY

Posturethroplasty SD is multifactorial and its true incidence is not known. Of all the factors, psychogenic causes seem to play a significant role and only the large-scale prospective trials, using validated questionnaires along with objective measurements, such as duplex ultrasonography, can clearly demonstrate the true incidence and causes of posturethroplasty SD. Even with current evidence suggesting the incidence to be low, de novo SD is a cause of major concern and anxiety among patients and surgeons alike and causes dissatisfaction even after a successful surgery. Due to its proximity to the cavernosal nerves and the pudendal arteries, bulbar urethroplasty has a higher likelihood of causing SD as compared with penile urethroplasty, but the evidence is sparse. As far as the nontransecting bulbar urethroplasty is concerned, there is not much controversy provided the precise indications prevail, but there are situations, like traumatic obliterated strictures, where there is no option other than to excise and perform anastomotic urethroplasty. PFUIs are associated with SD and any further deterioration posturethroplasty is unlikely and in some patients the function may even improve. PDE5Is are the first line of treatment and good response rates are noted in patients with urethral stricture or those with PFUI with neurogenic erectile dysfunction. Role of penile rehabilitation with PDE5I in PFUI is still considered investigational and further studies are required in this field.

REFERENCES

1. Andrich DE, Mundy AR. What is the best technique for urethroplasty? Eur Urol 2008;54:1031–41.

2. Rourke KF, Jordan GH. Primary urethral reconstruction: the cost minimized approach to the bulbous urethral stricture. J Urol 2005;173:1206–10.

3. Meeks JJ, Erickson BA, Granieri MA, et al. Stricture recurrence after urethroplasty: a systematic review. J Urol 2009;182:1266–70.

4. Erickson BA, Granieri MA, Meeks JJ, et al. Prospective analysis of erectile dysfunction after anterior urethroplasty: incidence and recovery of function. J Urol 2010;183:657–61.

5. Palminteri E, Berdondini E, De Nunzio C, et al. The impact of ventral oral graft bulbar urethroplasty on sexual life. Urology 2013;81:891–8.

6. Mundy AR. Results and complications of urethroplasty and its future. Br J Urol 1993;71:322.

7. Coursey JW, Morey AF, McAninch JW, et al. Erectile function after anterior urethroplasty. J Urol 2001;166:2273–6.

8. Sangkum P, Levy J, Yafi FA, et al. Erectile dysfunction in urethral stricture and pelvic fracture urethral injury patients: diagnosis, treatment, and outcomes. Andrology 2015;3:443–9.

9. Jackson MJ, Sciberras J, Mangera A, et al. Defining a patient reported outcome measure for urethral stricture surgery. Eur Urol 2011;60:60–8.

10. Patel DP, Elliott SP, Voelzke BB, et al. Patient-Reported Sexual Function After Staged Penile Urethroplasty. Urology 2015;86:395–400.

11. Barbagli G, De Angelis M, Romano G, et al. Long-term follow up of bulbar end-to-end anastomosis: a retrospective analysis of 153 patients in a single center experience. J Urol 2007;178:2470–3.

12. Blaschko SD, Sanford MT, Cinman NM, et al. De novo erectile dysfunction after anterior urethroplasty: a systematic review and meta-analysis. BJU Int 2013;112:655–63.

13. Blaschko SD, Sanford MT, Schlomer BJ, et al. The incidence of erectile dysfunction after pelvic fracture urethral injury: a systematic review and meta-analysis. Arab J Urol 2015;13:68–74.

14. Dogra PN, Saini AK, Seth A. Erectile dysfunction after anterior urethroplasty: a prospective analysis of incidence and probability of recovery–single-center experience. Urology 2011;78:78–81.

15. Yucel S, Baskin LS. Neuroanatomy of the male urethra and perineum. BJU Int 2003;92:624–30.

16. Barbagli G, De Stefani S, Annino F, et al. Muscle and nerve-sparing bulbar urethroplasty: a new technique. Eur Urol 2008;54:335–43.

17. Beysens M, Palminteri E, oosterlinck W, et al. Anastomotic repair versus free graft urethroplasty for bulbar urethral strictures: a focus on the impact of sexual function. Adv Urol 2015;2015:912438.

18. Erickson BA, Wysock JS, Mcvary KT, et al. Erectile function, sexual drive and ejaculatory function after reconstructive surgery for anterior urethral stricture disease. BJU Int 2007;99:607–11.

19. Xie H, Xu MY, Xu XL, et al. Evaluation of erectile function after urethral reconstruction: a prospective study. Asian J Androl 2009;11:209–14.

20. Xie H, Xu YM, Fu Q, et al. The relationship between erectile function and complex panurethral stricture: a preliminary investigative and descriptive study. Asian J Androl 2015;17:315–8.

21. Peterson AC, Webster GD. Management of urethral stricture disease: developing options for surgical intervention. BJU Int 2004;94:971–6.

22. Eltahawy EA, Virasoro R, Schlosemberg SM, et al. Long-term follow up for excision and primary anastomosis for anterior urethral strictures. J Urol 2007;177:1803–6.

23. Granieri MA, Webster GD, Peterson AC. Critical analysis of patient reported complaints and complications after urethroplasty for bulbar urethral stricture disease. Urology 2015;85:1489–93.

24. Morey AF, Kizer WS. Proximal bulbar urethroplasty via extended anastomotic approach–what are the limits? J Urol 2006;175:2145–9.

25. Ekerhult TO, Lindqvist K, Peeker R, et al. Low risk of sexual dysfunction after transection and non transection urethroplasty for bulbar urethral stricture. Urology 2013;190:635–8.

26. Jordan GH, Eltahawy EA, Virasoro R. The technique of vessel sparing excision and primary anastomosis for proximal bulbous urethral reconstruction. J Urol 2007;177:1799–802.

27. Palminteri E, Manzoni G, Berdondini E, et al. Combine dorsal plus ventral buccal muscosal graft in bulbar urethral reconstruction. Eur Urol 2008;83:81–90.

28. Palminteri E, Berdondini E, Florio M, et al. Two-sided urethra-sparing reconstruction combining dorsal preputial skin plus ventral buccal mucosa grafts for tight bulbar strictures. Int J Urol 2015;22:861–6.

29. Mundy AR. The treatment of sphincter strictures. Br J Urol 1989;64:626.

30. Blakely S, Caza T, Landas S, et al. Dorsal onlay urethroplasty for membranous urethral strictures: urinary and erectile functional outcomes. J Urol 2015;195(5):1501–7.

31. Bjurlin MA, Fantus RJ, Mellett MM, et al. Genitourinary injuries in pelvic fracture morbidity and mortality using the National Trauma Data Bank. J Trauma 2009;67:1033–9.

32. Harvey-kelly KF, Kanakaris NK, Eardley I, et al. Sexual function impairment after high energy pelvic fractures: evidence today. J Urol 2011;185:2027–34.

33. Shenfeld OZ, Kiselgorf D, Gofrit ON, et al. The incidence and causes of erectile dysfunction after pelvic fractures associated with posterior urethral disruption. J Urol 2003;169:2173–6.

34. Anger JT, Sherman ND, Dielubanza E, et al. Erectile function after posterior urethroplasty for pelvic

fracture-urethral distraction defect injuries. BJU Int 2009;104:1126–9.

35. Mark SD, Keane TE, Vandemark RM, et al. Impotence following pelvic fracture urethral injury: incidence, aetiology and management. Br J Urol 1995; 75:62–4.

36. Dhabuwala CB, Hamid S, Katsikas DM, et al. Impotence following delayed repair of prostate-membranous urethral disruption. J Urol 1990;144: 677–8.

37. Fu Q, Zhang J, Sa YL, et al. Recurrence and complications after transperineal bulboprostatic anastomosis for posterior urethral strictures resulting from pelvic fracture: a retrospective study from a urethral referral centre. BJUI 2013;112:E358–63.

38. Pratap A, Agarwal CS, Pandit RK, et al. Factors contributing to a successful outcome of combined abdominal transpubic perineal urethroplasty for complex posterior urethral disruptions. J Urol 2006; 176:2514–7.

39. El-Assmy A, Benhassan M, Harraz AM, et al. Ejaculatory function after anastomotic urethroplasty for pelvic fracture urethral injuries. Iny Urol Nephrol 2015;47:497–501.

40. Anger JT, Sherman ND, Webster GD. Ejaculatory profiles and fertility in men after posterior urethroplasty for pelvic fracture- urethral distraction defect injuries. BJU Int 2008;102:351–3.

41. Koraitim MM. On the art of anastomotic posterior urethroplasty: a 27-year experience. J Urol 2005; 173:135–9.

42. Morey AF, McAninch JW. Reconstruction of posterior urethral disruption injuries: outcome analysis in 82 patients. J Urol 1997;157:506–10.

43. Fu Q, Sun X, Tang C, et al. An assessment of the efficacy and safety of sildenafil administered to patients with erectile dysfunction referred for posterior urethroplasty: a single-center experience. J Sex Med 2012;9:282–7.

44. Sohn M, Hatzinger M, Goldstein I, et al. Standard operating procedures for vascular surgery in erectile dysfunction: revascularization and venous procedures. J Sex Med 2013;10:172–9.

45. Babaei AR, Safarinejad MR, Kolahi AA. Penile revascularization for erectile dysfunction: a systematic review and meta-analysis of effectiveness and complications. Urol J 2009;6:1–7.

46. Hellstrom WJ, Montague DK, Moncada I, et al. Implants, mechanical devices, and vascular surgery for erectile dysfunction. J Sex Med 2010;7:501–23.

47. Peng J, Yuan YM, Zhang ZC, et al. Daily low-dose tadalafil for erectile dysfunction induced by pelvic fracture urethral disruption. Zhonghua Nan Ke Xue 2013;19:443–5.

48. Tang YX, Gan Y, Zhang XB, et al. Low-dose tadalafil for erectile dysfunction following pelvic fracture-induced urethral injury: clinical observation of 42 cases. Zhonghua Nan Ke Xue 2013;19:539–41.

49. Feng C, Xu YM, Barbagali G, et al. The relationship between erectile dysfunction and open urethroplasty: a systematic review and meta-analysis. J Sex Med 2013;10:2060–8.

The Nontransecting Approach to Bulbar Urethroplasty

Stella Ivaz, MBBS, BMus (Hons), MA, MRCS, FRCS (Urol)[a],
Simon Bugeja, MD, MRCS (Ed), FEBU, MSC (Urol)[a],
Anastasia Frost, MSc (Urol), MBChB[a], Daniela Andrich, MD, MSc, FRCS[a],
Anthony R. Mundy, PhD (Hon) MS, FRCP, FRCS, FRACS (Hon)[a,b],*

KEYWORDS

• Urethral stricture • Urethroplasty • Urethral reconstruction

KEY POINTS

• The standard treatment for bulbar urethral strictures of appropriate length is excision and primary anastomosis (EPA), involving transection of the corpus spongiosum (CS).
• Recent evidence suggests there is a significant risk of sexual dysfunction and, potentially, of other adverse consequences as a result of transection of the CS.
• The authors have developed a technique of nontransecting anastomotic urethroplasty coupled with stricturoplasty, which seems to be just as effective as EPA.
• The authors also describe a stepwise "nontransecting approach" to all bulbar strictures, based on the cause of the stricture except those due to straddle injuries.
• EPA remains appropriate for strictures following straddle injuries.

INTRODUCTION

Most strictures in men arise in the bulbar urethra unless there is some obvious factor in the patient's history, such as pelvic trauma, or surgery for hypospadias, to indicate otherwise.[1–3] Iatrogenic strictures are common in the bulbar urethra, mainly due to catheterization or instrumentation, but the commonest group in the so-called developed world is described as "idiopathic," although some would regard them as congenital in origin[1,4–8]: an important point that will be discussed later.

Idiopathic strictures are generally short and sometimes only a membrane. They tend to be located at the junction of the proximal and middle thirds of the bulbar urethra (Fig. 1). When they first present, before any iatrogenic damage from instrumentation, they are associated with a minimal amount of fibrosis in the surrounding corpus spongiosum (CS).[9]

For many years, the surgical treatment of these patients, if they have failed to respond to first-line management by urethral dilatation or visual internal urethrotomy, has been excision of the stricture and end-to-end anastomosis, commonly known as excision and primary anastomosis or EPA.[10,11] This procedure has been reported to have a very high success rate and a very low incidence of side effects or complications,[10–13] but recent evidence and expert opinion suggest that there is a significant risk of potentially avoidable sexual dysfunction associated with the procedure.[14–18] This risk is attributed to transection of the CS.

Various authors, including the authors of this article, have observed that although EPA may be extremely effective (sexual dysfunction aside),

[a] Institute of Urology at UCLH, 16-18 Westmoreland Street, London W1g 8PH, UK; [b] UCLH NHS Foundation Trust, Trust Headquarters, 2nd Floor Central, 250 Euston Road, London NW1 2PG, UK
* Corresponding author. UCLH NHS Foundation Trust, Trust Headquarters, 2nd Floor Central, 250 Euston Road, London NW1 2PG, UK.
E-mail address: tony.mundy@uclh.nhs.uk

Urol Clin N Am 44 (2017) 57–66
http://dx.doi.org/10.1016/j.ucl.2016.08.012

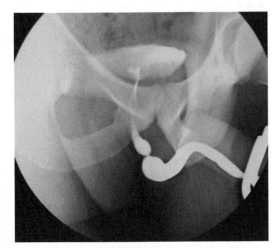

Fig. 1. Urethrographic appearance of a typical idiopathic stricture: typical in both length and location.

the amount of fibrosis excised with the stricture is actually very small, except after straddle injuries, and that the bulk of the CS, on transection, is healthy and, indeed, can bleed vigorously.[19–21] This observation casts doubt on the rationale for transection of the whole of the CS when only a small part of it is involved in the disease process.

In addition, Jordan and colleagues[19] noted that there are circumstances in which transection of the urethra may not be ideal, such as when a patient subsequently needs surgery for carcinoma of the prostate and develops postprostatectomy sphincter weakness incontinence for which he needs an artificial urinary sphincter to correct it, in which case the cuff of the artificial urinary sphincter and the effects of the previous EPA may compromise each other. They therefore developed an approach to proximal bulbar strictures to avoid transecting the urethra.[19,22]

The authors' own experience of approaching almost all longer bulbar strictures by a dorsal stricturotomy, with a view to patching them with a buccal mucosal graft (BMG), is that the stricture is usually easily visible on the inside of the urethra and not usually associated with much spongiofibrosis. Indeed, some strictures are so short that it is possible just to do a Heineke-Mickulicz type of stricturoplasty (HMS).[23,24] Hence, the authors were led, with strictures that were more than just a membrane but were still short enough to make it feasible, to try and excise the stricture and the associated spongiofibrosis intraurethrally (leaving the bulk of the CS intact) and simply restore epithelial continuity by stitching the epithelial margins together. The repair would then be completed by closing the dorsal stricturotomy incision with a stricturoplasty.

In 2012, the authors published their initial experience with this approach[18] and reported further follow-up data and their increasing experience since.[25–27] The authors have stressed that this is "an approach." The fundamental premises have been that bulbar strictures are usually short and that there is little in the way of spongiofibrosis except after straddle injury—in which case excision and end-to-end anastomosis would be appropriate. Otherwise, the authors approach the stricture surgically in the same way in all patients. They mobilize the bulbar urethra, perform a dorsal stricturotomy, and then inspect the urethra from the inside. If the stricture is amenable to local excision and repair of the stricture intraurethrally, the authors do so or otherwise do a dorsal patch urethroplasty, usually using a BMG as described by Barbagli,[28,29] and now more properly, if less precisely, described as an augmented bulbar urethroplasty.[30]

This review describes and updates the authors' experience with such an approach, including the development of an augmented nontransecting technique to deal with more complex bulbar strictures.

PATIENTS AND METHODS

Between January 2009 and December 2014, the authors performed 405 bulbar urethroplasties, excluding staged repairs and perineal urethrostomies. Seventy-two of these were standard EPA procedures, in other words, transecting in the traditional way. Fifty-eight of these 72 patients had suffered straddle injuries of the bulbar urethra, and the remaining 14 patients were either revisional cases or had developed gross fibrosis as a result of infection. In almost all cases, the need for an EPA could be predicted from the patient's clinical features and imaging.

Of the remaining 333 patients, 232 had a relatively long stricture, usually as a result of or made worse by instrumentation, and were treated by a dorsal buccal mucosal graft patch urethroplasty (DBMGPU) **(Fig. 2)**. The other 101 patients had relatively shorter strictures, usually idiopathic and without so much previous instrumentation. They had a dorsal stricturotomy and a stricturoplasty, or a nontransecting excision of the stricture and a stricturoplasty or an augmented nontransecting approach,- as described in later discussion. As with the "EPA group," the dorsal stricturotomy approach in these 333 patients was almost always predictable preoperatively even though the exact procedure could only be decided by the operative findings, as described in later discussion.

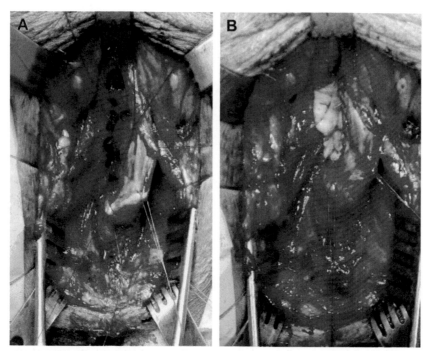

Fig. 2. DBMGPU. (*A*) The stricturotomy. Note the diathermy burns to control bleeding from the perforators. (*B*) The dorsal BMG patch quilted onto the tunica albuginea (over the diathermy burns).

All patients complete a Patient Recorded Outcome Measure (PROM) questionnaire[31,32] and have a urinary flow study and an ascending urethrogram and micturating cystogram preoperatively. Postoperatively, they have a PROM and a flow study at 3 months, 6 months, and 1 year and annually thereafter with urethrography at 1, 2, and 5 years.

All of these patients have had a minimum of 18 months' follow-up within which time any recurrence could reasonably be expected to be radiologically demonstrable if not clinically apparent.[33]

SURGICAL PROCEDURES
Preparation

In all cases, the patient is placed in the low (sometimes called "social") lithotomy position.[34,35] The legs are supported with Allen Yellofin stirrups. Elasticated stockings, inflatable leggings, and low-molecular-weight heparin are used to minimize the risk of deep vein thrombosis. Antibiotic prophylaxis with gentamicin and coamoxiclav is started at induction of anesthesia and is followed by a second dose later the same day.

Incision and Mobilization

After skin preparation and draping, a floppy-tipped Terumo guidewire is passed up the urethra, through the stricture, and into the bladder. The bulbar urethra is then exposed and mobilized through a midline perineal incision.[34] It is fully mobilized from its dorsal attachment to the tunica albuginea of the corpora cavernosa all the way proximally to the perineal membrane and distally as far as the attachment of the suspensory ligament of the penis to the shaft of the penis. The posterior attachment of the proximal third of the urethra to the perineal body is left intact to avoid damage to bulbar arteries (**Fig. 3**).

After adequate mobilization of the bulbar urethra, a dorsal stricturotomy is made onto the tip of a 20-French catheter placed to abut against the distal end of the stricture, and stay stitches are placed to hold the bulbar urethra open at this point so that there is a clear view of the guidewire running into the stricture. A stricturotomy is then performed using either tenotomy scissors or Potts scissors, or, occasionally, a scalpel. The bulbar urethra proximal to the stricture is then opened up into normal-caliber urethra for a further 1–2 cm and further stay stitches are place to hold the proximal urethra open. There should now be a clear view of the stricture and of the normal-caliber urethra on either side (**Fig. 4**).

An assessment can now be made of the length of the stricture, the degree of fibrosis, and the stretchability of the bulbar urethra as judged by the ability to bring the 2 ends of the stricturotomy

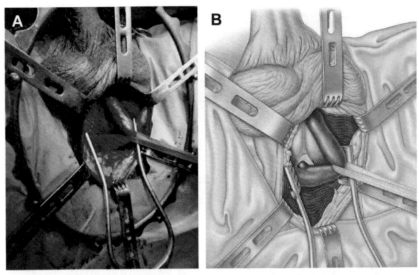

Fig. 3. Exposure: (*A*) operative photograph; (*B*) diagrammatic representation.

together without tension for a horizontal closure of the suture line. These findings, together with the preoperative radiological imaging, allow a judgment to be made as follows:

1. The stricture is very short, perhaps only a membrane, with minimal spongiofibrosis, and a stricturoplasty is possible. Or, at the other extreme:
2. The stricture and the adjacent normal-caliber urethra are worse than predicted on preoperative imaging and the 2 ends of the stricturotomy cannot be brought together without tension for a stricturoplasty type of closure, so only a DBMGPU is feasible. Or:
3. The stricture is somewhere in between these 2 extremes of length and is amenable to

intraurethral excision and mucosal anastomosis to restore epithelial continuity and then a stricturoplasty-type of closure. Or:

4. The stricture may be too long for option 3 and DBMGPU may seem the obvious answer, but there is an obliterative segment that is best excised because patch urethroplasties are less successful in the presence of an obliterative segment.[1,21,36] The obliterative segment is therefore excised and the defect closed, either by direct suture or by grafting with oral mucosa if it is too long be closed by direct suture. The dorsal stricturotomy is then closed by an oral mucosal graft (usually BMG), as in a DBMGPU, rather than by a stricturoplasty.

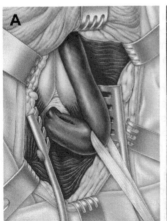
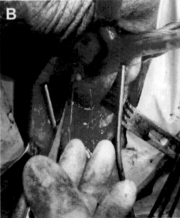
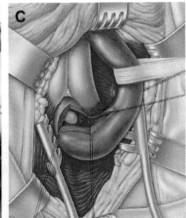

Fig. 4. Dorsal stricturotomy: (*A*) the incision; (*B*) operative photograph after placing the stay sutures; (*C*) diagrammatic representation. There is a catheter in the proximal urethra to demonstrate the lumen more clearly.

Stricturoplasty (Heineke-Mickulicz Type of Stricturoplasty)

A stricturoplasty is performed according to the general principles of the Heinecke-Mickulicz procedure.[23,24] In other words, the longitudinal stricturotomy is closed transversely (**Fig. 5**), hence, the importance of the stretchability of the bulbar urethra to allow the 2 ends of the longitudinal stricturotomy to be brought together as the center of the transverse closure. Interrupted 5-0 Vicryl sutures are used: usually one in the dorsal midline and 2 on either side. These sutures are full-thickness sutures; one must verify that the epithelium is picked up with every pass of the needle. It is often easier to place the sutures first and then tie them parachute style afterward rather than to place them and tie them one at a time. It is sometimes helpful to open the intercrural plane at the root of the penis to create more space within which to work.

Nontransecting Excision of the Stricture and Mucosal Anastomosis

If the stricture is more than just a membrane, then it is excised together with the underlying fibrosis, and the mucosal ends are stitched together with 4 to 6 interrupted 5-0 Vicryl sutures (**Fig. 6**). The urethra is then closed with an HMS, as above.

Augmented Nontransecting Excision of the Stricture and Mucosal Anastomosis

If the stricture is obliterative or has a (near) obliterative segment, then that segment is excised and the defect closed, either by direct suture or by grafting with oral mucosa if it is too long be closed by direct suture (**Fig. 7**), and a dorsal BMG patch is used to close the urethra.

Results

In total, the authors have treated 101 patients with HMS, nontransecting excision of the stricture and mucosal anastomosis (NTABU), or augmented nontransecting excision of the stricture and mucosal anastomosis (ANTABU). Sixteen patients have had an HMS alone; 57 patients have had an NTABU (including an HMS), and 28 patients have had an ANTABU.

Thus far, with a minimum of 18 months' follow-up, there have been only 2 recurrent strictures demonstrable radiologically, giving a success rate of 99 of 101 (99%). There has been erectile dysfunction beyond 6 months in 2 patients (2%): one after an NTABU and the other after an ANTABU. This incidence is substantially less than the incidence of 18% to 23% associated with EPA.[12–16] There has been an incidence of postmicturition dribbling of 2 of 16 (13%) in the HMS group, 5 of 57 (18%) in the NTABU group, and 7 of 29 (24%) in the ANTABU group: the same incidence as the authors find in their patients who have had a straightforward dorsal patch urethroplasty. Three patients have had a satisfactory radiological result (no residual or recurrent stricture), but an unsatisfactory symptomatic result because of urodynamically proven detrusor failure.

In short, the authors have the same sort of success rate with the nontransecting approach as with the transecting approach and with an

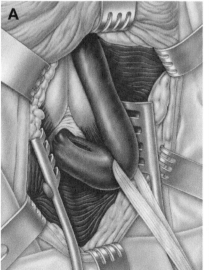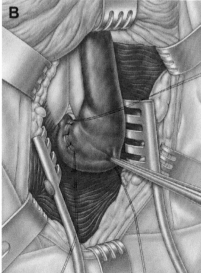

Fig. 5. Transverse closure of stricturotomy incision: HMS: (*A*) the original longitudinal stricturotomy; (*B*) The transverse closure.

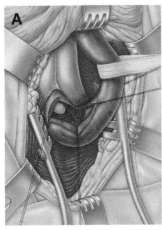
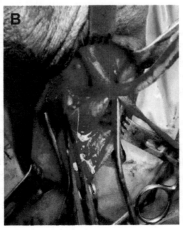
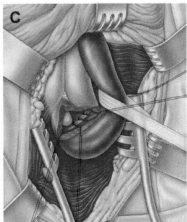

Fig. 6. (*A*) Stricture excised exposing the healthy spongiosum beneath (diagram) and urethra sutured; (*B*) operative photograph; (*C*) diagrammatic representation.

incidence of side effects or complications, which is at least the same if not better but, potentially, with less long-term morbidity because of the preservation of the CS. Whether this proves to be a definite advantage will only be shown in longer-term studies. At this stage, the authors are not trying to show that the nontransecting approach is superior to the standard approach, only that it is at least equivalent, but also that it follows the general trend in surgical practice to minimize bleeding and surgical trauma as much as possible.

DISCUSSION

What the authors have described here is a stepwise approach to the management of nontraumatic

bulbar urethral strictures and the way in which this approach has been developed. Having excluded straddle injuries and various unusual problems rarely seen in patients presenting for surgery for the first time, the authors approach the stricture in all patients through a dorsal stricturotomy. Having made a detailed visual assessment, they then treat very short strictures by stricturoplasty; short strictures by excision, mucosal anastomosis, and stricturoplasty; intermediate-length strictures and those with obliterative segments by augmented nontransecting urethroplasty; and long strictures by a "traditional" dorsal patch urethroplasty (**Fig. 8**).

The key to this technique is that the proximal bulbar urethra is not surrounded by the CS on its dorsal aspect (**Fig. 9**). Indeed, strictly speaking,

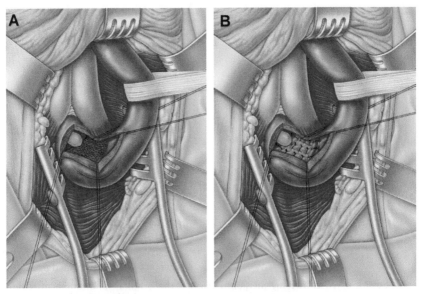

Fig. 7. (*A*) Stricture excised and (*B*) BMG quilted on to the raw spongiosum.

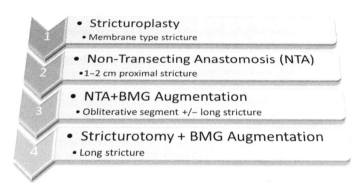

- **Stricturoplasty**
  - Membrane type stricture
- **Non-Transecting Anastomosis (NTA)**
  - 1–2 cm proximal stricture
- **NTA+BMG Augmentation**
  - Obliterative segment +/– long stricture
- **Stricturotomy + BMG Augmentation**
  - Long stricture

Fig. 8. The stepwise approach to nontransecting urethroplasty after a dorsal stricturotomy.

anatomically,[37,38] this segment is part of the membranous urethra but below the perineal membrane, meaning that a dorsal stricturotomy at this site does not damage the blood flow through the CS through which all the blood supply to the urethra is derived. Furthermore, when the DBMGPU is performed, the tunica albuginea is a very satisfactory bed for the graft—arguably (but debatably) more so than the CS is for a ventral patch

procedure—because although both tissues are well vascularized to act as a bed for a graft, the tunica albuginea is more stable and more resilient. Finally, in most patients, there is a very satisfactory view of the inside of the bulbar urethra through this approach, which allows for excision of the stricture and the related spongiofibrosis except when surgical access is impaired as in extreme obesity, hip disease, or some other problem.

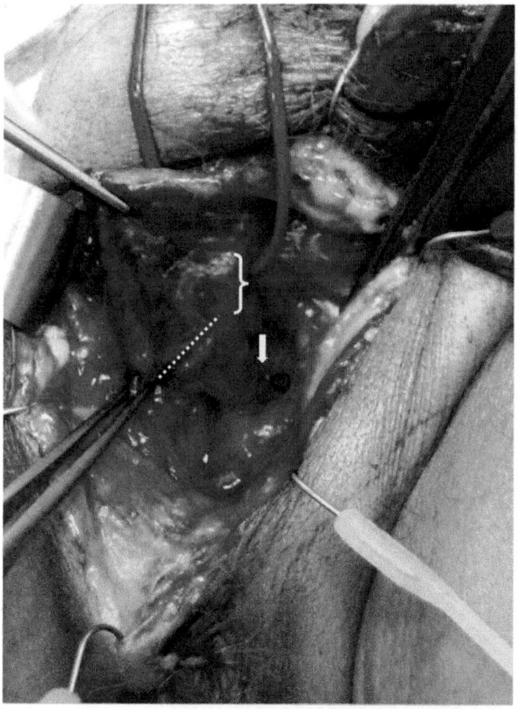

The other potentially important point about avoiding urethral transection is that the arterial blood supply of the urethra may be compromised in certain circumstances. The authors have mentioned a hypothetical example of a patient who may at some stage require implantation of an artificial sphincter. A more practical problem is the patient with hypospadias who requires a bulbar urethroplasty for a coexisting bulbar stricture. This problem is not uncommon. Indeed, in the authors' experience, some 15% of patients with hypospadias require bulbar urethral surgery at some stage in adolescence or adult life.[1] The exact nature of this coincidental stricture is debatable. In some, it may be as a consequence of instrumentation or previous surgery for the hypospadias. In others, it may be a coincidental idiopathic stricture particularly if this type of idiopathic stricture might prove to be congenital in origin.

The arterial supply of the urethra has 4 components (**Fig. 10**).[39] The principal component is thought to be the bulbar artery on each side, which arises from the pudendal artery deep in the perineum. Second in importance is the retrograde blood flow that comes ultimately from the common penile artery, via the dorsal artery of the penis, into the glans, and then retrogradely back through the CS to the bulb. Third, there are circumflex branches from the dorsal artery of the penis that run round the shaft of the penis at about 1-cm intervals through to the urethra deep to Buck fascia. Finally, there are perforating vessels directly

Fig. 9. Cadaveric dissection of the bulbomembranous urethra. The arrow indicates the anterior margin of the perineal membrane; the *dotted line* indicates the original relationship of the urethra to the perineal membrane, and the brackets indicate that part of the urethra below the perineal membrane that is not covered by the spongiosum on its dorsal aspect. The CS is retracted by the 2 pairs of forceps.

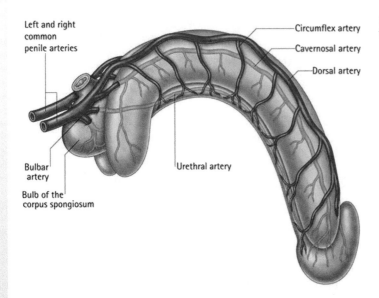

Fig. 10. The arterial blood supply of the urethra, CS, and corpora cavernosa.

Left and right common penile arteries

Circumflex artery

Cavernosal artery

Dorsal artery

Bulbar artery

Urethral artery

Bulb of the corpus spongiosum

through the tunica albuginea directly into the body of the CS and the urethra on either side of the dorsal midline. These perforators are rarely, if ever, mentioned in the literature, but they are a significant feature during urethral mobilization (see **Fig. 2**A). In hypospadias, the blood flow through the bulbar arteries, the circumflex branches, and the penetrating branches may all be intact, but the retrograde flow through the CS might be impaired because of hypoplasia of the glans and of the distal CS. How often this has an impact on the blood flow within the bulbar urethra is not known, but it is certainly, at the very least, a risk factor for relative ischemia of the bulbar urethra, giving a nontransecting approach of potentially substantial advantage.

Of equal importance with the urethral vasculature is the cause of the stricture, as the authors have alluded to by their repeated reference to the need to identify urethral trauma due to straddle injury and treat these patients differently because of the dense transmural traumatic fibrosis (**Fig. 11**). Arguably, these should not be described as strictures because the abnormality is so

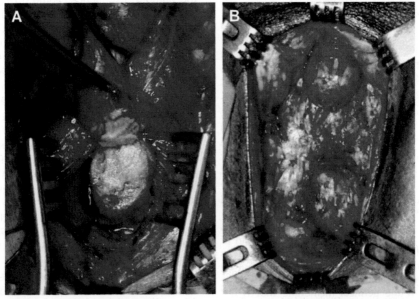

Fig. 11. Urethral strictures after straddle injuries. (*A*) Typical full-thickness spongiofibrosis during transection. (*B*) Complete necrosis and segmental defect.

different. Indeed, by contrast, idiopathic strictures are short, almost membranelike constrictions with little if any associated fibrosis unless this is induced iatrogenically by a surgeon by performing a urethrotomy or dilatation. It is almost true that idiopathic = very short and very short = idiopathic, particularly at that specific point of the junction of the proximal and middle thirds of the bulbar urethra (see **Fig. 1**).

In all other strictures, ischemia is a significant factor, typically associated with aging, and after endoluminal trauma, associated with catheterization and instrumentation, hence, presumably, the tendency for these to be longer strictures that have a life-long tendency to recur,[40] particularly in patients with microvascular disease such as diabetics and cigarette smokers.

These points are important because whether idiopathic strictures are indeed congenital, they are certainly different from iatrogenic and ischemic strictures because of the minimal fibrosis and normality of the urethra on either side. The group of patients with idiopathic strictures is therefore the group in whom a permanent cure is truly possible, whereas in all other patients their (current) stricture may just be the (current) local manifestation of a stricture-prone urethra. Given that urethrotomy and dilatation are usually not curative[41] and tend to make any fibrosis worse and any stricture longer,[42] the almost universal tendency to continue with these treatments in patients with idiopathic strictures is unjustifiable, except when poor general health makes palliation justifiable, because they risk making a curable stricture incurable.

In this review, the authors have concentrated on the intraurethral excision of the stricture and the mucosal anastomosis, if only to stress that transection of the urethra, and of the CS in particular, is not necessary. It is important however not to understate the importance of the stricturoplasty. It is not just a means of closing the stricturotomy; it is an integral part of the repair as a whole because it has been in urethroplasty procedures described several times over the years[43–46] and not just in urology.[24] It is also in keeping, of course, with the general concept of spatulation of any anastomosis to reduce the risk of recurrent stenosis.

SUMMARY

In conclusion, although the standard approach to bulbar urethral strictures of appropriate length by EPA gives excellent results in competent hands, it is unnecessary, except in patients with transmural fibrosis or frank necrosis as a consequence of trauma or gross infection. In most circumstances bulbar strictures have comparatively small amounts of spongiofibrosis and can be treated by intraurethral excision and mucosal anastomosis with stricturoplasty or even just stricturoplasty alone with results that are just as satisfactory.

At this stage, the results of the "nontransecting approach" show equivalence with EPA. The authors will need longer-term follow-up to see whether equivalence is sustained in practice. The authors will also see whether this approach is superior in patients with hypospadias and impaired retrograde blood flow within the CS, or those who have had a bulbar urethroplasty by a transecting approach who subsequently need implantation of an artificial urinary sphincter, for example, In any case, it seems to the authors sensible to try and restrict the trauma during urethroplasty (or indeed any surgical procedure) as far as possible.

REFERENCES

1. Mundy AR, Andrich DE. Urethral strictures. BJU Int 2011;107:6–26.
2. Fenton AS, Morey AF, Aviles R, et al. Anterior urethral strictures: etiology and characteristics. Urology 2005;65:1055–8.
3. Lumen N, Hoebeke P, Willemsen P, et al. Etiology of urethral stricture disease in the 21st century. J Urol 2009;182:983–7.
4. Netto NR, Martucci RC, Goncalves ES, et al. Congenital stricture of male urethra. Int Urol Nephrol 1976;8:55–61.
5. Donnellan SM, Costello AJ. Congenital bulbar strictures occurring in three brothers. Aust N Z J Surg 1996;66:423–4.
6. Cobb BG, Wolf JA Jr, Ansell JS. Congenital stricture of the proximal urethral bulb. J Urol 1968;99:629–31.
7. Moorman JG. Congenital anomalies of the urethra. Br J Urol 1968;40:636–9.
8. Narborough GC, Elliot S, Minford JE. Congenital stricture of the urethra. Clin Radiol 1990;42:402–4.
9. Cavalcanti AG, Costa WS, Baskin LS, et al. A morphometric analysis of bulbar urethral strictures. BJU Int 2007;100:397–402.
10. Eltahawy EA, Virasoro R, Schlossberg SM, et al. Long-term follow-up for excision and primary anastomosis for anterior urethral strictures. J Urol 2007;177:1803–6.
11. Terlecki RP, Steele MC, Valadez C, et al. Grafts are unnecessary for proximal bulbar reconstruction. J Urol 2010;184:2395–9.
12. Morey AF, Watkin N, Shenfeld O, et al. SIU/ICUD consultation on urethral strictures: anterior urethra - primary anastomosis. Urology 2014;83(3 Suppl):S23–6.

13. Santucci RA, Mario LA, McAninch JW. Anastomotic urethroplasty for bulbar urethral stricture: analysis of 168 patients. J Urol 2002;167:1715–9.

14. Barbagli G, Sansalone S, Romano G, et al. Bulbar urethroplasty: transecting vs. nontransecting techniques. Curr Opin Urol 2012;22:474–7.

15. Barbagli G, Guazzoni G, Lazzeri M. One-stage bulbar urethroplasty: retrospective analysis of the results in 375 patients. Eur Urol 2008;53:828–33.

16. Al-Qudah H, Santucci R. Buccal mucosa onlay urethroplasty versus anastomotic urethroplasty (AU) for short urethral strictures: which is better? J Urol 2006; 175:103 [abstract: 313].

17. Erickson BA, Granieri MA, Meeks JJ, et al. Prospective analysis of erectile dysfunction after anterior urethroplasty: incidence and recovery of function. J Urol 2010;183:657–61.

18. Palminteri E, Franco G, Berdondini E, et al. Anterior urethroplasty and effects on sexual life: which is the best technique? Minerva Urol Nefrol 2010; 62:371–6.

19. Jordan GH, Eltahawy EA, Virasoro R. The technique of vessel sparing excision and primary anastomosis for proximal bulbous urethral reconstruction. J Urol 2007;177:1799–802.

20. Andrich DE, Mundy AR. Non-transecting anastomotic bulbar urethroplasty: a preliminary report. BJU Int 2012;109(7):1090–4.

21. Welk BK, Kodama RT. The augmented nontransected anastomotic urethroplasty for the treatment of bulbar urethral strictures. Urology 2012;79:917–21.

22. Gur U, Jordan GH. Vessel-sparing excision and primary anastomosis (for proximal bulbar urethral strictures). BJU Int 2008;101:1183–95.

23. Mickulicz-Radecki J. Zur operativen Behandlung des stenosirenden Magengeschwures. Arch Klin Chir 1888;37:79–90.

24. Pocivavsek L, Efrati E, Lee KYC, et al. Three-dimensional geometry of the Heineke-Mikulicz strictureplasty. Inflamm Bowel Dis 2013;19:704–11.

25. Mundy AR, Andrich DE. Non-transecting bulbar urethroplasty. In: Brandes SB, Morey AF, editors. Advanced male urethral and genital reconstructive surgery. New York: Humana Press; 2014. p. 531–40.

26. Bugeja S, Andrich DE, Mundy AR. Non-transecting bulbar urethroplasty. Transl Androl Urol 2015;4:41–50.

27. Bugeja S, Ivaz S, Frost AV, et al. Non-transecting bulbar urethroplasty using buccal mucosa. Afr J Urol 2016;22:47–53.

28. Barbagli G, De Angelis M, Romano G, et al. Long-term followup of bulbar end-to-end anastomosis: a retrospective analysis of 153 patients in a single center experience. J Urol 2007;178:2470–3.

29. Andrich DE, Leach CJ, Mundy AR. The Barbagli procedure gives the best results for patch urethroplasty of the bulbar urethra. BJU Int 2001;88:385–9.

30. Latini JM, McAninch JW, Prandes SB, et al. Epidemiology, etiology, anatomy and nomenclature of urethral stenoses, strictures and pelvic fracture urethral disruption injuries. Urethral strictures. An international consultation on urethral strictures. Marrakech (Morocco), October 13–16, 2010. Jordan G, Chapple C, Heyns C, editors. Societe Internationale d'Urologie. 2012. p. 1–7.

31. Jackson MJ, Sciberras J, Mangera A, et al. Defining a patient-reported outcome measure for urethral stricture surgery. Eur Urol 2011;60:60–8.

32. Jackson MJ, Chaudhury I, Mangera A, et al. A prospective patient-centred evaluation of urethroplasty for anterior urethral stricture using a validated patient-reported outcome measure. Eur Urol 2013; 64:777–82.

33. Meeks JJ, Erickson BA, Granieri MA, et al. Stricture recurrence after urethroplasty: a systematic review. J Urol 2009;182:1266–70.

34. Mundy AR. Anastomotic urethroplasty. BJU Int 2005; 96:921–44.

35. Andrich DE, Mundy AR. Complications of "social" lithotomy. BJU Int 2010;106(Suppl 1):40–1.

36. Gingu C, Dick A, Patrascoiu S, et al. Nontransecting augmented roof anastomosis: the technique of choice for long bulbar urethral strictures with limited spongiofibrosis. Eur Urol Suppl 2014;13:e77.

37. Davies DV, Davies F, editors. The male urethra. Ch. in: Gray's anatomy. 33rd edition. London: Longmans; 1962. p. 1516.

38. Federative Committee on Anatomical Terminology. Terminologia anatomica. Stuttgart (Germany): Thieme; 1998. p. 70.

39. Juskiewenski S, Vaysse PH, Moscovici J, et al. A study of the arterial blood supply to the penis. Anat Clin 1982;4:101–7.

40. Andrich DE, Dunglison N, Greenwell TJ, et al. The long-term results of urethroplasty. J Urol 2003;170:90–2.

41. Santucci R, Eisenberg L. Urethrotomy has a much lower success rate than previously reported. J Urol 2010;183:1859–62.

42. Greenwell TJ, Castle C, Andrich DE, et al. Repeat urethrotomy and dilation for the treatment of urethral stricture are neither clinically effective nor cost-effective. J Urol 2004;172:275–7.

43. Stern M. A plastic operation for the cure of urethral stricture. JAMA 1920;74:85–8.

44. Young HH, Davis DM. Operations on the urethra. In: Young HH, Davis DM, editors. Young's practice of urology. Philadelphia: WB Saunders; 1926. p. 565–642. Chapter 20.

45. Cabot H. Plastic operations for epispadias, hypospadias and urethral stricture. Mayo Clin Proc 1930;5:315–6.

46. Duckett JW. MAGPI (meatoplasty and glanuloplasty): a procedure for subcoronal hypospadias. Urol Clin North Am 1981;8:503–12.

Management of Panurethral Stricture

Sanjay Kulkarni, MD, Jyotsna Kulkarni, FRCS, Sandesh Surana, MD, Pankaj M. Joshi, MD*

KEYWORDS

- Urethra • Panurethral • Full-length • Stricture • One-stage • Complex

KEY POINTS

- Panurethral structure is a complex and challenging issue.
- Staged urethroplasty was preferred in past.
- Lichen sclerosus is a genital skin disease, and staged urethroplasty.
- Single-stage buccal graft procedures have an advantage over staged procedures and flaps.
- Multicenter published review concludes that panurethral structure treated in most high-volume centers with a single-stage dorsal onlay buccal graft augmentation urethroplasty has superior results over staged urethroplasty or flap procedures.

 Video content accompanies this article at http://www.urologic.theclinics.com.

URETHROPLASTY FOR PANURETHRAL URETHRAL STRICTURE

Introduction

The surgical treatment of urethral strictures varies according to cause, location, and length of stricture. Treatment of strictures involving the bulbar urethra is relatively well defined. However, management of long-segment urethral stricture, or panurethral stricture disease, is challenging, and the literature on the subject is not abundant.

Panurethral stricture involves the full length of the urethra from meatus until the most proximal bulb. The incidence of panurethral strictures is increasing. Most panurethral strictures in the Indian subcontinent are due to lichen sclerosus. Iatrogenic causes are also on the increase. Iatrogenic causes include urethral catheterization, cystourethroscopy, transurethral resection, and previous urethral surgeries.

Review of literature suggests the use of staged Johanson's urethroplasty and the use of flaps for these complex patients. Because lichen sclerosus is a disease of genital skin, local skin flaps or staged urethroplasty is best avoided because the disease can recur in the tubularized urethra. The late 1990s saw the revolution of buccal mucosa urethroplasty. Subsequently panurethral strictures started being treated with augmentation using buccal grafts. The authors present the management algorithm for panurethral strictures (**Fig. 1**).

Evaluation of Patient

Symptomatic stricture disease usually presents with decreased flow associated with other lower urinary tract symptoms. Patients may have recurrent urinary tract infections. Usually strictures with lichen sclerosus have a long-standing history. Iatrogenic strictures tend to present early. Significant numbers of iatrogenic strictures are nearly obliterative in nature, and the patient could be referred with a suprapubic tube.

Many patients have a history of direct visual internal urethrotomy and dilatations. Uroflowmetry, ultrasonography, and cystourethroscopy are

No Conflict of Interest.

Kulkarni Reconstructive Urology Center, 3, Rajpath Society, Paud Road, Pune 411038, India

* Corresponding author. Kulkarni Reconstructive Urology Center, 3, Rajpath Society, Opp Vanaz Engineering One No 5, Paud Road, Pune 411038, India.

E-mail addresses: drpankajmjoshi@gmail.com; kesi95@gmail.com

Urol Clin N Am 44 (2017) 67–75

http://dx.doi.org/10.1016/j.ucl.2016.08.011

0094-0143/17/© 2016 Elsevier Inc. All rights reserved.

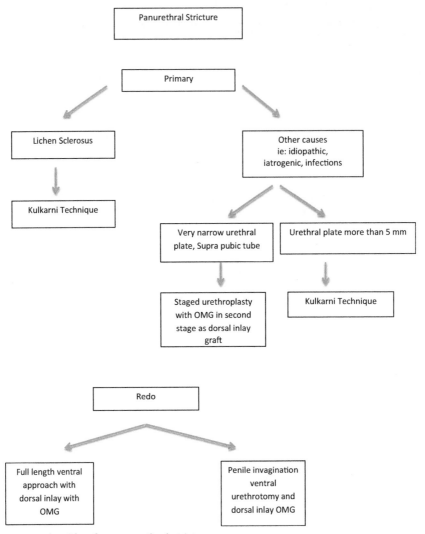

Fig. 1. Management algorithm for panurethral strictures.

important adjuncts in the diagnosis of panurethral stricture disease. Ultrasonography is done to evaluate upper tract. Retrograde urethrography (**Fig. 2**) and voiding cystourethrography determines the location, length, and severity of the stricture. It is important to note that the membranous urethra does not have spongiosum and is almost never involved in panurethral stricture. However, the bulbar urethra may be involved up to the bulbomembranous junction.

SURGICAL TECHNIQUES OF PANURETHRAL REPAIRS
Johanson's Staged Urethroplasty

The classic 2-stage method was developed in the 1950s by Bengt Johanson.[1] The Johanson

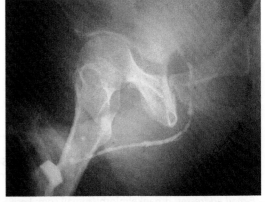

Fig. 2. Urethrogram in a patient with panurethral stricture.

procedure is based on marsupialization of the structured urethra, followed by a second surgical stage approximately 4 to 6 months after the first stage has healed. In the past, scrotal or perineal skin was used for urethral reconstruction. The great achievement of Johanson's technique was its use in all types of strictures, apart from initiating an era of urethral reconstructive surgery. The drawbacks of this technique resulted from the use of hair-growing scrotal and perineal skin, which leads to chronic urinary tract infection, abscesses, stone formation, fistulation, sacculation, and diverticula formation in the reconstructed urethra.

In the 1980s, Schreiter and Noll[2,3] reported a 2-stage mesh graft procedure in an attempt to avoid the use of scrotal or perineal skin by using a hairless skin graft, which is transferred in a 2-stage procedure. Although this technique can be used in every type of stricture, apparently its best indication is in complex strictures, especially associated with severe tissue scarring and absence of healthy penile skin for urethral reconstruction.

Flaps

Several flaps have been described and used in panurethral stricture reconstruction. Quartey from Ghana described a penile fasciocutaneous skin flap in 1983.[4] It is so called because the incision on the penis resembles the letter Q. The Q flap is outlined with the penis on stretch and the penis degloved, meticulously preserving the blood supply on the tunica dartos pedicle. The Q-flap is sewn into place after ventral urethrotomy as an onlay flap with running absorbable suture. The fossa navicularis is typically reconstructed through a glans-wings or a glans-preserving technique. Once the pendulous portion of the onlay flap is sewn in, the patient in repositioned into the lithotomy position, the flap is transferred to the perineum through a scrotal tunnel wide enough to accommodate loose passage of the flap.

In 1993, McAninch described the circular fasciocutaneous penile flap for the reconstruction of extensive urethral stricture.[5] Circular fasciocutaneous penile flap originates on the distal penis and uses Buck's fascia as the major vascular supply. He reported his results with the use of this flap for 1-stage reconstruction of complex anterior urethral strictures involving long penile and also bulbar urethral strictures in 66 men.[6] The stricture length measured up to 24 cm (average 9.08 cm). The flap was used as an onlay procedure and tubularised flap for urethral substitution. In some cases, additional adjunctive tissue transfer and proximal graft placement was required. Initial

success rate was 79%, rising up to 95% after an additional procedure. Recurrent strictures occurred usually at the proximal and distal anastomotic sites. The penile circular fasciocutaneous flap reliably provided 12–15 cm of length for reconstruction in most patients, even though approximately 90% had been previously circumcised. The less favorable results were seen in patients after flap tubularization for urethral replacement. Because of compartment syndrome noted in 2 different cases due to prolonged exaggerated lithotomy position (usually occurs if the patient remains in this position more than 5 hours), the authors begin the operation with flap harvesting with the patient in the supine position, thereby reducing exposure to the lithotomy position by 2-3 hours.

The potential major advantage of these flap procedures is to allow a single-stage reconstruction of long-segment and complex strictures and to avoid the need for additional, morbid, time-consuming tissue transfer techniques.

These two procedures require plastic surgery training. A common complication with the above two flaps, particularly with inexperienced surgeons, is necrosis of penile skin proximal to the flap.[6–8] In some instances, this penile skin necrosis may lead to wound infection and ultimately to disruption of the flap and necrosis.

Major challenge of flaps is the meticulousness needed to preserve the pedicle and blood flow without causing necrosis to the remaining penile skin. Not many urologists are trained in plastic surgical techniques. Lichen sclerosus is a disease of genital skin. If penile skin flap is used in reconstruction of urethra the risk of failure is very high. In Staged urethroplasty what is essentially tubularised is the penile skin and again this technique cannot be used in Lichen sclerosus. Best suited option which can be used in all patients with panurethral strictures is oral mucosa graft augmentation urethroplasty.

The use of grafts in urethral reconstruction has become a popularized surgical option worldwide. They are quick and relatively easier to harvest and deploy. The widespread popularity of oral mucosa in urethral reconstruction has similarly allowed the introduction of new techniques in long-segment and panurethral stricture repair.

Single-Staged Buccal Graft Urethroplasty

Staged reconstructions are associated with significant inconvenience to some patients, exposing them to an increased risk of morbidity due to multiple general anesthetics. In addition, revision is common after 2-stage operations, and in one series, half of the patients ended up needing a 3-stage repair. Kulkarni and colleagues[9–11] published a pioneering technique of single-stage augmentation urethroplasty using oral mucosa graft (OMG) through a perineal incision (Video 1).

The patient is nasally intubated, and 2 teams work simultaneously at the donor and recipient site, with separate sets of instruments. The oral mucosa is harvested from both cheeks as described by Kulkarni and colleagues.[9] The patient is placed in simple lithotomy position, with heels carefully placed in Yellofin stirrups (Allen Medical Systems, Acton, MA, USA) and no pressure on the calves, to avoid peroneal nerve injury. The suprapubic, scrotal, and perineal skin is shaved, disinfected using chlorhexidine, and draped. Preoperatively, urethroscopy is performed using a 6-French rigid ureteroscope. A 3-French guidewire is inserted. Methylene blue is injected into the urethra, and a midline perineal incision is made. The bulbar urethra is dissected, only on the left side of patient, from the corpora cavernosa. The bulbospongiosus muscle and central tendon of the perineum are left intact ventrally. The dorsal aponeurosis of the bulbospongiosus is approached by dissecting around the muscle and incised, allowing access to the dorsal urethra (**Fig. 3**A). The dissection is taken across the midline. On the right, the urethra remains attached to the corpora cavernosa for its full length, preserving its neurovascular supply.

Invaginating the penis into the incision (**Fig. 3**b), the penile urethra is similarly dissected off the corpora cavernosa along the left side, to the coronal sulcus (**Fig. 4**). The urethra is rotated, exposing the dorsal surface, and opened longitudinally (**Fig. 5**). A wide dorsal meatotomy is performed externally (**Fig. 6**). The first OMG is sutured to the dorsal apex of the meatus (**Fig. 7**), pushed into the penile urethra, spread and fixed to corpora cavernosa over the midline. Another OMG is applied to the corpora cavernosa opposite the bulbar urethra. Continuous upward traction is applied to the inverted penis while applying the penile graft to prevent chordee. The grafts are 1.5 cm in width; they are spread and fixed with quilting sutures (**Fig. 8**). The OMG margin is sutured to the (patient's) right side of the urethral plate, and a 14-French silicone catheter is inserted. The full length of urethra is rotated back to its original position over the graft. Continuous 4-0 polyglactin suture is used to stabilize the urethral margins onto corpora cavernosa on the left (**Fig. 9**). The dorsal aponeurosis of bulbospongiosus is then closed. Colles fascia, perineal fat, and skin are closed with interrupted absorbable sutures. The catheter is maintained for 4 weeks (**Fig. 10**).

Postoperative Care and Follow-Up Criteria

The patient ambulates on postoperative day 1 and is usually discharged 2 days after surgery. All patients receive postoperative broad-spectrum antibiotics and oral antibiotics till the catheter is removed. The authors do not perform pericatheter

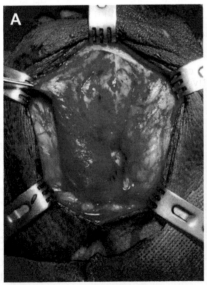
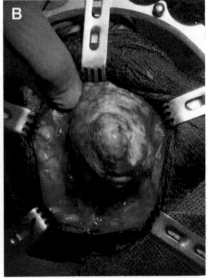

Fig. 3. (*A*) One-sided dissection of bulbar urethra. The proximal two-thirds of the bulbospongiosus are left intact. The distal one-third of the bulbospongiosus, which attaches to the corpus cavernosum, is incised. (*B*) Penis is invaginated by incising the fascia over the urethra, with left hand pushing the penis down to the perineum.

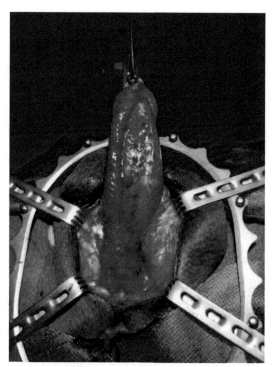

Fig. 4. One-sided dissection of the entire anterior urethra.

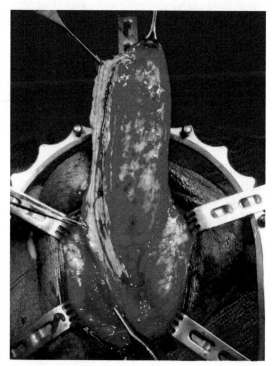

Fig. 5. Urethra opened along dorsal aspect longitudinally.

urethrogram for all cases. It is done for redo urethroplasty and is performed 4 weeks postoperatively, and if no leak, the catheter is removed. The patient performs uroflowmetry at 3, 6 and 9 months postoperatively and then annually, or sooner if clinically indicated. If the patient experiences a decreased force of stream and uroflowmetry less than 12 mL/s, further investigation is undertaken, including urethrography, urethral ultrasound, and urethrocystoscopy.

Due to the global referral base and to reduce patients travel we prefer to use the internet for follow up. Patients follow up with their referring urologist to get their uroflowmetry which is then communicated using email, Whatsapp and other internet based applications.

Management of panurethral strictures with Kulkarni technique is standardized. Most patients with panurethral strictures undergo this single-stage surgery.

The study is an observational, descriptive, retrospective, and prospective analysis in 318 consecutive male patients. Inclusion criteria were fit men ranging from 20 to 76 years of age with panurethral strictures. The average stricture length varied from 10 to 19 cm. Most patients were referred by other urologists. Referrals included patients with primary or failed urethroplasty. Patients with history of retention or referred with suprapubic catheters were considered obliterative.

All patients were treated by five reconstructive urologists in the unit which also included Fellows using 1-stage OMG urethroplasty through a perineal incision. In January 2016, all data related to patients from June 1995 to June 2015 were retrospectively and prospectively collected and analyzed.

The primary outcome measure was success of surgery, and the secondary end point was the treatment of failures.

Clinical outcome was considered a failure when any instrumentation was necessary, including dilation. Uroflowmetry was performed every 3 months the first year and annually thereafter. Patients with symptomatic poor flow less than 12 mL/s and urinary tract infections were evaluated with uroflowmetry, urethrography, urethral ultrasound, and urethroscopy.

RESULTS

A total 318 patients were eligible for review according to the inclusion/exclusion criteria. Median patient age was 44.6 years (range 20–76). The overall median follow-up was 59 months (range 6.4–192). The cause of stricture was lichen sclerosus in 184 patients (57.86%). The mean stricture

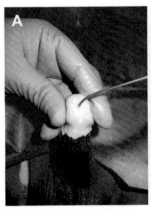
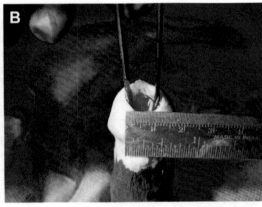

Fig. 6. (*A*) Initial meatus. (*B*) After dorsal meatotomy.

length was 14 cm, with a range of 10 to 19 cm. Of 318 patients, 283 (88.99%) had no previous urethral surgery, and 35 (11.01%) had undergone previous failed urethroplasty.

Of the 318 patients, 270 (84.90%) were successful and 48 (15.10%) were failures. Of the 283 patients who had no prior surgery, 244 (89.39%) were successful and 39 (11.61%) failed. In the group of 35 redo urethroplasty patients, 20 (57.85%) had a successful outcome and 15 (42.15%) failed.

Of the 48 patients with recurrent strictures, no patient had a full-length recurrence. When a stricture recurred, it was at the proximal end of the graft, the junction of 2 grafts, or the meatus. The recurrences generally manifest as a nonobliterative fibrous ring. The failed patients were managed with interval dilation, repeat urethroplasty, meatotomy, and perineal urethrostomy. Repeat urethroplasty after failure was performed by OMG patch placement ventrally for the proximal bulbar urethra.

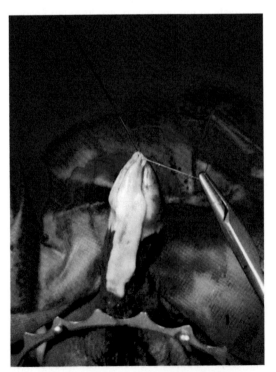

Fig. 7. Securing the graft at the apex of meatus.

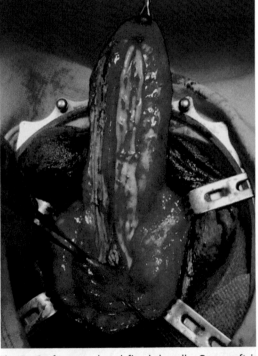

Fig. 8. Grafts spread and fixed dorsally. One graft is opposite the penile urethra, and one graft is opposite the bulbar urethra.

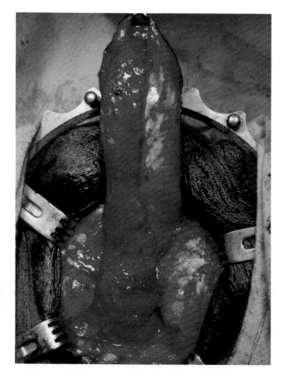

Fig. 9. Urethra rotated back into position over the grafts.

49 of 318 patients had obliterative strictures based on the authors' definition of history of retention or suprapubic catheters. The success rate of one urethroplasty in obliterative strictures is 57.1%, and 60.3% of obliterative strictures were due to iatrogenic cause.

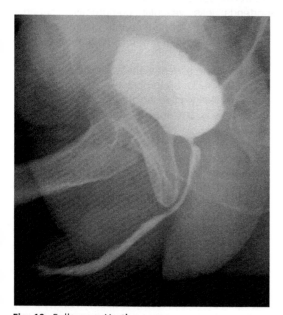

Fig. 10. Follow up Urethrogram.

Surgical Technique of Redo Panurethral Urethroplasty

It is common in the authors' tertiary referral center to perform redo single-stage urethroplasty for panurethral strictures. The approach to such cases depends on previous surgeries. If previously staged Johanson's urethroplasty was performed, it is challenging to invaginate penis. The possibility of penile invagination can be judged by feeling the skin over the underlying urethra. In such complex patients, a ventral urethrotomy is performed, and the urethra is opened across the full length from meatus until the most proximal bulbar urethra. A midline incision is made in the urethral plate. OMG are harvested and inserted as dorsal inlay across the full length of the urethra. The augmented urethra is then tubularized, and second layer closure is performed with dartos tissue.

Another approach is the minimally invasive Kulkarni approach of penile invagination through perineal incision. Assuming that previous urethroplasty was performed with a dorsal approach, it is challenging to mobilize the urethra dorsally again. Hence, the urethra is incised ventrally across the full length of the urethra, and dorsal inlay OMG urethroplasty is performed.

DISCUSSION

Panurethral strictures by definition involve the whole anterior urethra and form a complex subset of urethral stricture disease. Lichen sclerosus remains a primary cause for panurethral stricture disease, particularly in the Asian subcontinent. Recently, there has been a trend toward more iatrogenic panurethral strictures. Prolonged catheterization or traumatic catheterization results in panurethral stricture secondary to inflammation and ischemia of the urethra. Another proposed mechanism includes local allergic reaction to the catheter or lubricant used at time of placement. Endoscopic instrumentation of the urethra, particularly with transurethral resection of the prostate, can also lead to urethral trauma and ischemia, resulting in stricture formation. Aside from technical considerations (obvious catheter trauma or complicated procedures), it remains difficult to identify those at higher risk for panurethral stricture.

Historically, 2-stage urethroplasty was favored for the management of panurethral strictures. The Johanson's 2-stage technique, first described in 1953, involves buried epithelium (originally local skin, which later evolved to autologous graft) based on the Denis-Browne principle.[1] Upon review of the literature, several institutions have experimented with other tissue-transfer techniques, including fasciocutaneous skin flap with or without simultaneous use of buccal mucosa graft,[7,12] or tunica albuginea.[13] There has been a long-standing view of using 2-stage urethroplasty for panurethral strictures. The primary concern with the 2-stage Johanson's technique is that it relies on genital skin for the neo-urethra. As was shown in the authors' series, more than 50% of panurethral strictures are secondary to lichen sclerosus. Any 2-stage procedure with genital skin will have a high risk of recurrence secondary to incorporation of diseased skin in urethra. Due to this reason that the authors developed a single-stage urethroplasty for panurethral stricture.

DEVELOPMENT OF KULKARNI TECHNIQUE

Kulkarni performed urethrectomy for bladder cancer using penile invagination during his training in the United Kingdom. Panurethral strictures were mainly treated by 2-stage procedures until the 1990s. Dorsal onlay buccal graft urethroplasty was popularized by Barbagli in 1996. Kulkarni performed dorsal onlay buccal graft urethroplasty for panurethral strictures in India. The penile urethra was approached through circumcision incision and bulbar urethra through perineal incision. The penoscrotal junction would be a watershed area with technical difficulty. To avoid this problem, Kulkarni applied the penile invagination technique and performed dorsal onlay buccal graft urethroplasty for panurethral incision through the perineum. By invagination, the full anterior urethra was now visualized as a single unit. The concept of meatotomy with graft insertion from meatus until proximal bulb was now possible through a single incision in the perineum. Initially, the urethra was mobilized circumferentially. Barbagli and Kulkarni[10] published the techniques of muscle-sparing bulbar urethroplasty. The one-side dissection technique was then amalgamated, with the Kulkarni technique further refining it. Today, the technique consists of single-stage, penile invagination, one-side dissection, dorsal onlay buccal graft urethroplasty. This approach also opened up the avenue of treating penile urethral strictures without incision on penis. This approach is now widely followed across reconstructive urology units.

Dubey and colleagues[14] reported their experience comparing the 1-stage Kulkarni technique and 2-stage repairs for panurethral strictures secondary to lichen sclerosus. They concluded that 1-stage procedures had better success, and although staged procedures could be successful, they were fraught with technical difficulties and multiple revisions.[14] Although the Johanson staged repair has fallen out of favor as first-line therapy, it can still be used to salvage the most complex urethral strictures.[15]

In a very recent transcontinental multi-institutional study, Warner and colleagues[16] reported the complication rates of different surgical techniques to repair long-segment and panurethral strictures. The complication rate was higher in the fasciocutaneous cohort compared with those without a flap (32% vs 14%, respectively; $P = .02$). In this review, a 2-stage Johanson urethroplasty was not as successful as the buccal mucosal graft procedure (BMG) (64% vs 82.5%, respectively). It was found that 2-stage Johanson urethroplasties performed with skin had a higher failure rate than those performed with a BMG (66.7% recurrence rate vs 28.3%, respectively). Flaps have higher complication rates as compared with one-stage urethroplasty.[1] Fasciocutaneous single stage OMG augemntation (Kulkarni technique) had superior results.

Oral mucosal grafts are now considered the standard substitution material for urethral surgery. Surgical procedures involving oral mucosa have better success rates and less morbidity compared with fasciocutaneous flaps.

The 1-stage Kulkarni technique offers several key advantages. The perineal approach avoids a penile incision and suture line, minimizing the risk of urethrocutaneous fistula. Penile cosmesis is excellent, with no hypospadiac meatus, and reduces the incidence of chordee. Functionally, this technique preserves the bulbospongiosus muscle, urethral neurovascular supply, and the central tendon of the perineum. Kulkarni technique portends less vascular compromise, superior muscular support of the urethra, decreased post-micturition dribbling, and preservation of ejaculatory function.[9,10,17]

In the authors' series, the success rates for primary and redo urethroplasty were significantly different, likely reflecting the severity of the disease process, and fibrosis after the previous failed repair.

Recurrences after panurethral stricture repair often occur at either the meatus, the junction of the 2 buccal mucosa grafts, or the proximal anastomosis. The authors attempt to minimize meatal recurrence by performing a wide dorsal meatotomy. At our institution, recurrences at the meatus are managed with ventral meatotomy. Recurrence at the junction of the 2 grafts is first treated by one attempt at urethrotomy/dilation, followed by dorsal inlay buccal mucosa graft (Asopa technique). Proximal recurrence is similarly treated with one attempt of urethrotomy/dilation, followed by ventral onlay buccal mucosa graft urethroplasty.

The authors attempt to adhere to a strict follow-up regimen for patients undergoing panurethral urethroplasty. Patients are followed at 3, 6, 9, and 12 months, and annually thereafter with clinical history, physical examination, and uroflowmetry. If they are unwilling or unable to travel, the authors ask the primary urologist to perform the follow-up. Diminished flow on uroflowmetry is further investigated with retrograde urethrogram and cystoscopy. Low flows (Qmax 10–13 mL/s) may be attributed to stricture recurrence, benign prostatic hyperplasia, or bladder hypotonicity. The authors attempt to avoid overinvestigation in patients who report good flow and improvement in symptoms.

SUMMARY

- Panurethral stricture disease is a complex disease.
- One-stage repairs with BMG offer an excellent option for patients with long-segment and panurethral stricture disease.
- In cases of lichen sclerosus, 1-stage BMG has better outcomes than a 2-stage repair.
- In cases with obliterative or absent urethral plate due to non–lichen sclerosus cause, a 2-stage Johanson urethroplasty with BMG augmentation offers a viable alternative.
- No surgical technique should compromise penile length, cause chordee, and affect cosmesis.
- The Kulkarni technique for panurethral urethroplasty is minimally invasive, with excellent postoperative outcomes, improved cosmesis, and excellent functional outcomes.

ACKNOWLEDGMENTS

We would like to acknowledge the help of Dr Devang J Desai in editing the manuscript.

SUPPLEMENTARY DATA

Supplementary data related to this article can be found at http://dx.doi.org/10.1016/j.ucl.2016.08.011.

REFERENCES

1. Johanson B. Reconstruction of the male urethra in strictures. Acta Chir Scand 1953;167(Suppl):1.
2. Schreiter F, Noll F. Mesh graft urethroplasty. World J Urol 1987;5:41–6.
3. Schreiter F, Noll F. Mesh graft urethroplasty using split-thickness skin graft or foreskin. J Urol 1989; 142:1223–6.
4. Quartey JK. One-stage penile/preputial cutaneous island flap urethroplasty for urethral stricture: a preliminary report. J Urol 1983;129(2):284–7.
5. Martins FE, Kulkarni SB, Joshi P, et al. Management of long segment and panurethral stricture disease [review]. Adv Urol 2015;2015:853914.
6. McAninch JW. Reconstruction of extensive urethral strictures: circular fasciocutaneous penile flap. J Urol 1993;149:488–91.
7. McAninch JW, Morey AF. Penile circular fasciocutaneous skin flap in 1-stage reconstruction of complex anterior urethral strictures. J Urol 1998;159: 1209–13.
8. Dubey D, Kumar A, Bansal P, et al. Substitution urethroplasty for anterior urethral strictures: a critical appraisal of various techniques. BJU Int 2003;91: 215–8.
9. Kulkarni S, Barbagli G, Kirpekar D, et al. Lichen sclerosus of the male genitalia and urethra: surgical options and results in a multicenter international experience with 215 patients. Eur Urol 2009;55:945.
10. Kulkarni S, Barbagli G, Sansalone S, et al. One-sided anterior urethroplasty: a new dorsal only graft technique. BJU Int 2009;104:1150.
11. Kulkarni SB, Barbagli G. One-sided anterior urethroplasty: a new dorsal onlay graft technique. J Urol Suppl 2010;183:e593 [abstract: V1537].
12. Buckley JC, McAninch JW. Distal penile circular fasciocutaneous flap for complex anterior urethral strictures. BJU Int 2007;100:221.
13. Mathur RK, Sharma A. Tunica albuginea urethroplasty for panurethral strictures. Urol J 2010;7: 120.
14. Dubey D, Sehgal A, Srivastava A, et al. Buccal mucosal urethroplasty for balanitis xerotica obliterans related urethral strictures: the outcome of 1 and 2-stage techniques. J Urol 2005;173:463.
15. Al-Ali M, Al-Hajaj R. Johanson's staged urethroplasty revisited in the salvage treatment of 68 complex urethral stricture patients: presentation of total urethroplasty. Eur Urol 2001; 39:268.
16. Warner JN, Malkawi I, Dhradkeh M, et al. A multi-institutional evaluation of the management and outcomes of long-segment urethral strictures. Urology 2015;85(6):1483–7.
17. Barbagli G, De Stefani S, Annino F, et al. Muscle- and nerve-sparing bulbar urethroplasty: a new technique. Eur Urol 2008;54:335.

Effect of Lichen Sclerosis on Success of Urethroplasty

Michael A. Granieri, MD, Andrew C. Peterson, MD*,
Ramiro J. Madden-Fuentes, MD

KEYWORDS

- Lichen sclerosis • Urethroplasty • Urethral stricture • Balanitis xerotica obliterans
- Perineal urethrostomy

KEY POINTS

- Lichen sclerosis is a chronic inflammatory skin disease with a variable presentation commonly affecting the anogenital area in both men and women.
- Management of urogenital lichen sclerosis is predicated on the extent of disease.
- Most patients can be treated with conservative therapies consisting of minimally invasive surgical techniques and potent topical steroids.
- Surgical intervention may be indicated when the disease process is extensive or recalcitrant to conservative therapy.
- Perineal urethrostomy is an attractive option with high patient satisfaction for extensive urethral lichen sclerosis in patients who are unwilling or unfit for 2-stage repair.

INTRODUCTION

Lichen sclerosis (LS), previously termed balanitis xerotica obliterans, is a chronic inflammatory skin disease commonly affecting the anogenital area in both men and women. In 1976, the International Society for the Study of Vulvovaginal Disease concluded that the terminology LS should be adopted for men and women.[1] In men, it commonly manifests in excess of simple balanitis, hence the accepted change in terminology. The presentation of LS in both men and women is variable and ranges from a focal disease process to an extensive degree of involvement presenting in childhood or adulthood. It may extend beyond the glans penis and affect the penile shaft skin, urethral meatus, and urethra.[2,3] Consequently, the diverse presentation means diverse treatment is necessary with variable success rates. A higher predilection of LS in women compared with men is well established. Urethral involvement of LS is largely seen in men, however.[4] The extent of urethral disease may be limited to the urethral meatus or progress to panurethral involvement.

In this article, the authors describe the presentation, pathogenesis, epidemiology, and their current management algorithm for male patients with LS.

PRESENTATION

Genital involvement with LS may present with local pruritus, dysuria, phimosis, paraphimosis, fissures, whitish skin, and bothersome lower urinary tract symptoms (LUTS) when the urethra is involved (**Fig. 1**). Riddell and colleagues[5] reported

Disclosure Statement: There are no conflicts of interest. No sources of external funding to be reported.
Division of Urology, Department of Surgery, Duke University Medical Center, DUMC 3146, Durham, NC 27710, USA
* Corresponding author.
E-mail address: Drew.Peterson@duke.edu

Urol Clin N Am 44 (2017) 77–86
http://dx.doi.org/10.1016/j.ucl.2016.08.004
0094-0143/17/© 2016 Elsevier Inc. All rights reserved.

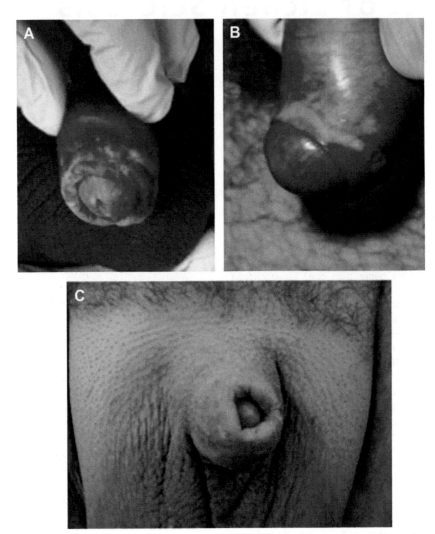

Fig. 1. Variable presentation of LS. (*A*) Whitish discoloration, with foreskin fissuring and glanular irritation. (*B*) Phimosis, skin thinning, glanular and preputial irritation. (*C*) Buried penis, penile entrapment, dense scarring.

common symptoms in patients diagnosed with LS. Tight foreskin was noted in 25.8%, pruritus in 18%, painful erections in 13.6%, and cracking and bleeding in 9.1%. Up to 19.7% of patients reported difficulty passing urine, which raises concern for either meatal or urethral involvement. Chronic inflammatory changes may be associated with genital ulceration and superimposed infections. Significant scarring and genital deformation may be noted as a consequence.

PATHOGENESIS

LS is characterized microscopically by the presence of hyperkeratosis, thinning of the epidermis, loss of rete pegs, and collagen deposition in the dermis (**Fig. 2**). A histiocytic or lymphocytic infiltrate is also noted and has led to the theory of an

inflammatory cause.[6,7] A variety of precipitating factors, including autoimmune processes, infections, and trauma, have also been suggested to contribute to the development of LS.

Autoimmunity

Immune-related dysregulation has been suggested as the cause of LS. Histopathologic findings of abnormal T-cell clones in the lymphocytic infiltrate of tissue affected by LS argue for autoimmune dysregulation as the underlying factor leading to pathogenesis.[8] Attempts at identification of a putative antigen suggest that extracellular matrix protein 1 (ECM1) may play a role. Initially, this was suggested by the overlapping dermatologic clinical and histologic findings between lipoid proteinosis and LS. Lipoid proteinosis is an

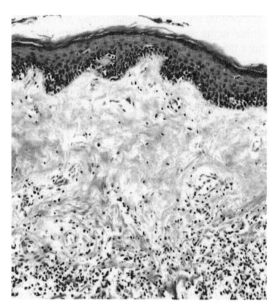

Fig. 2. Skin diseased by LS (hematoxylin-eosin, original magnification ×100). Loss of rete pegs, collagen deposition, lymphocytic infiltrate are all noted.

autosomal-recessive genetic disorder leading to loss of function of ECM1. Circulating antibodies to ECM1 have been noted in a higher proportion of patients with LS than controls.[9] Debate still remains whether these circulating antibodies are due to exposure of the site-specific antigens from another inciting event, or whether circulating antibodies are the cause of the genital skin changes.

In addition, other studies have also suggested a genetic susceptibility and autoimmune basis to LS. Bjekic and colleagues,[10] in a case control study of 73 patients with LS, noted an association between the presence of LS and prior genital injury, vitiligo, family history of alopecia areata, and thyroid gland disease. Azurdia and colleagues[6] compared a cohort of biopsy-proven LS patients with controls and found an increased frequency of class II HLA antigens DR11, DR12, and DQ7, suggesting an immunopathogenesis for this disease.

Infection

An infectious pathogen has been suggested as a potential driving factor for LS based on histologic evaluation of skin biopsies. A few studies have linked spirochetes, *Borrelia burgdorferi*, and acid-fast bacilli to LS.[11,12] However, others have attempted to confirm these findings and have failed to demonstrate a correlation in specimens of LS.[13,14] At the current time, the authors think that the evidence does not support infection as the cause of LS.

Trauma

The Koebner phenomenon is described as dermal lesions arising from trauma and has been suggested as a cause for LS.[15] Various reports suggest the development of LS after circumcision at suture lines as well as following sunburns and radiation therapy.[4,16,17] It remains unclear if these events herald the development of the immunopathogenesis resulting in LS in susceptible patients.

Degeneration to Malignancy

Importantly, LS is a relapsing and progressive disease with reported degeneration to squamous cell carcinoma (SCC). However, a direct causation has not been reliably described. Most reports have identified LS changes in the background of SCC. No published prospective cohort of patients diagnosed with LS has been reported to then ascertain the incidence of subsequent SCC.

Depasquale and colleagues[18] reported 522 men surgically treated for LS and noted a 2.3% rate of associated SCC. In this cohort, the indication for surgery was SCC and LS was a secondary finding. Given that many of the patients were referred for surgical treatment of SCC, these data do not necessarily suggest LS as a precursor to SCC. There are other reports associating LS with SCC. Barbagli and colleagues[19] reported 130 men with surgically treated LS and noted an 8.4% rate of premalignant or malignant histopathological features on re-review of the pathologic specimens. Similarly, of 20 patients with confirmed penile carcinoma, Powell and colleagues[20] noted that 50% of those patients had SCC in a background of LS. Last, Velazquez and Cubilla[21] reported 68 patients with known SCC and found LS in 33% of the specimens. The authors have longitudinally followed a cohort of men with biopsy-proven LS. Of 68 patients with biopsy-proven LS followed for a mean of 36 months, there were no instances of development of SCC or premalignant lesions.[22] To the authors' knowledge, this is the only report to date that has longitudinally followed patients with biopsy-proven LS.

The current data are unclear regarding the role of LS in the subsequent development of SCC. Although the authors' experience has not demonstrated degeneration to malignancy, longer follow-up interval with a larger number of patients will provide further insight into this critical question.

EPIDEMIOLOGY

The true prevalence of LS in men is likely underreported, because many affected individuals will have minimally symptomatic disease. In children presenting with phimosis for circumcision, pathologic analysis has shown that LS may be present in up to 20% to 30% of patients.[23–25] An estimated 28% of men seen in an outpatient clinic diagnosed with LS by physical examination were asymptomatic.[5] In 1971, Wallace[26] reported an estimated prevalence of LS between 1 in 300 and 1 in 1000 in a cohort of men referred to a community-based dermatology clinic. The age of presentation has been reported highest in the third and fourth decade of life.[27] However, in a large cohort of Department of Defense beneficiaries, the age distribution was more than double in the fourth and fifth decade of life compared with the first 3 decades. The highest prevalence was seen in men greater than 61 years old.[28]

Management of urogenital LS is predicated on the extent of disease, and because of its variable presentation, this ranges from conservative therapy to surgical intervention. Depasquale and colleagues[18] reported 428 men with LS as the primary disease process. In this cohort, 70.1% of patients had LS involving only the foreskin and glans, 4.9% the urethral meatus, and 20% the urethra. In patients with disease limited to the foreskin or glans circumcision, topical therapies may be sufficient. However, in cases of severe glanular, meatal, or urethral involvement, more aggressive surgical therapies are necessary.

EVALUATION FOR PENILE/URETHRAL DISEASE

Although the diagnosis of LS is often from history and physical examination (see **Fig. 1**; **Fig. 3**), several skin disorders, such as scleroderma, penile intraepithelial neoplasia (previously known as erythroplasia of Queyrat and Bowen disease),

leukoplakia, and Zoon balanitis, may present with similar signs and symptoms. Therefore, the authors think a confirmatory biopsy is imperative to rule out malignant and premalignant penile lesions and further guide therapy.[4] Moreover, because the external manifestations of LS do not accurately predict the degree of urethral involvement, they recommend a LUTS evaluation in all patients.

In those patients with self-reported LUTS or with an elevated American Urological Association Symptom Index score, a retrograde urethrogram is the study of choice to evaluate for urethral involvement (**Fig. 4**). In addition, cystoscopy can be performed, usually revealing a narrowed urethral lumen with pale mucosa. The presence of atypical cystoscopic findings, such as significant desquamation, focal nodular narrowing, and ulcerated or bleeding mucosa, may signify malignant transformation and warrant a biopsy.

Urethral involvement of LS usually results from proximal progression of meatal LS. However, Liu and colleagues[29] reported in a cohort of 70 patients with isolated bulbar urethral stricture disease that almost 26% of men had histologic findings diagnostic of LS with no evidence of distal involvement. In this cohort, patients with LS on reexamination of the abnormality tended to have a previous failed intervention.[29] In a large observational study, Palminteri and colleagues[30] reported 1439 men undergoing urethroplasty. Of these patients, 193 (13.4%) were due to LS. Penile urethral strictures due to LS occurred in 107 patients, panurethral in 69 patients, and anterior urethral (penile and bulbar) in 17 patients. Interestingly, no isolated instances of LS and bulbar strictures were noted. Similarly, Barbagli and colleagues[31] reported 925 patients with a history of urethral

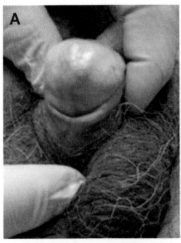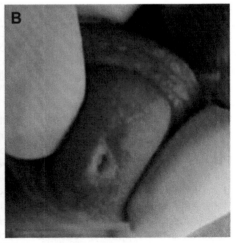

Fig. 3. (*A*) Glanular and (*B*) meatal involvement with LS.

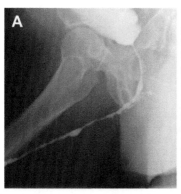
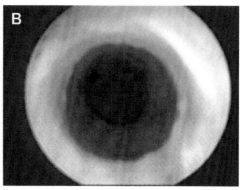

Fig. 4. (*A*) Retrograde urethrogram in patient with LS and evidence of biopsy-proven panurethral stricture disease. (*B*) Cystoscopy of patient with LS demonstrating an irregular lumen with concentric white scar bands consistent with LS. Tissue is normally friable and minimally pliable.

stricture disease undergoing urethral reconstruction and found LS as the cause in 14% of the patients.

Although these studies do indicate that skip lesions and isolated urethral lesions are possible, the authors have not observed this in their practice. Regardless, these findings merit consideration when managing isolated bulbar urethral strictures because of the higher risk of recurrence in patients with LS.

MANAGEMENT OF GENITAL LICHEN SCLEROSIS

The 3 overarching goals of management are alleviation of symptoms, prevention and treatment of urethral stricture disease, and prevention and detection of malignant transformation. In their practice, the authors have developed 3 additional goals to also address improving quality of life:

1. Unobstructed voiding
2. Painless intercourse
3. Adequate cosmesis[32]

As a result, the authors have shifted their paradigm in the management of LS. Most patients can be treated with minimally invasive therapies, including high-potency steroids and self-calibration before embarking on potentially morbid and invasive surgical interventions.[33]

Most patients afflicted by LS can be treated with conservative therapies before surgical intervention (**Fig. 5**). Classically, LS involving the foreskin, glans, and meatus can initially be managed by a short course of topical steroids. In the authors' practice, clobetasol propionate 0.05% topical application provides resolution of many of the bothersome presenting symptoms.

Kyriakou and colleagues[34] reported a 90.2% success rate in treatment with newly diagnosed,

biopsy-proven genital LS in a cohort of 41 men. There were statistically significant improvements in patient-reported outcomes and objective physician measures with the use of clobetasol proprionate 0.05% cream for 8 weeks. Long-term sequelae of LS were not assessed, but the authors' treatment goals focus on symptom relief and prevention of disease progression. Tausch and Peterson[35] reported a subgroup of patients with LS involving only the penile foreskin and glans, who were treated with an aggressive combination of clobetasol ± circumcision. In this subgroup, no recurrences were noted on long-term follow-up (mean of 44.2 months).

Classically, urethral involvement of LS is managed surgically. However, Potts and colleagues[33] recently reported a cohort of men with biopsy-proven LS and urethral stricture disease managed with intraurethral steroids with excellent results. In this cohort, an intraurethral steroid regimen consisting of self-calibration twice daily for 3 months with a clobetasol-lubricated catheter resulted in a success rate of 89%. Furthermore, no patients in the series progressed to requiring formal surgical intervention. The promising results of this approach provide a significant minimally invasive option for urologists and patients alike before consideration of formal surgical intervention.

Surgical intervention is still needed when the disease process is extensive, bothersome, or recalcitrant to conservative therapy. In a series of 287 patients, Depasquale and colleagues[18] demonstrated that 92% of men with foreskin or glans involvement had a long-term cure with circumcision alone. In their practice, the authors have noted that circumcision alone may alleviate mild glans changes obviating further therapy.

Meatal stenosis and distal urethral strictures secondary to LS may be treated with topical

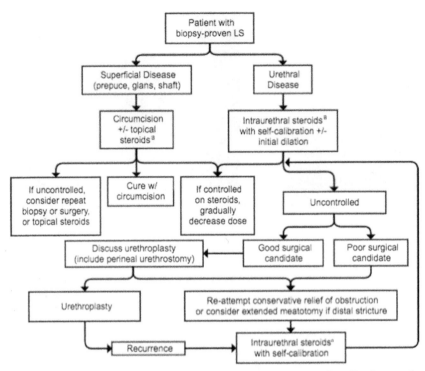

Fig. 5. Updated algorithm for management of biopsy-proven LS in men. [a] Steroid application BID for 2–3 months. BID, twice a day.

steroids, intermittent self-calibration, or surgical intervention, including urethral reconstruction with buccal grafts or extended meatotomy. When an extended meatotomy is performed, the penis will have a hypospadic appearance. Excellent success with extended meatotomy has been reported for complex fossa navicularis and distal strictures. In a cohort of 16 patients with distal strictures who underwent extended meatotomy, success rates were as high as 87%.[36] The cause of these strictures was not described; however, Tausch and Peterson[35] reported outcomes of extended meatotomy in patients with known LS. Of the 12 patients treated, there were no recurrences identified.

Morey and colleagues[36] described the use of a first-stage Johanson technique to perform an extended meatotomy in patients with distal urethral strictures. In this technique, the meatus is open ventrally until healthy patent mucosa is noted and easily calibrated with a 24-Fr bougie à boule. The edges are marsupialized with absorbable suture (**Fig. 6**).

Distal urethroplasty in the management of urethral stricture disease resulting from LS is typically performed with a substitution urethroplasty technique rather than a fasciocutaneous flap approach due to the high failure rate of the latter. Venn and Mundy[37] reported outcomes of 12 patients with

LS who underwent a local pedicle flap distal urethroplasty. They report 100% failure in these patients and advocate against the use of fasciocutaneous flaps for this disease process. Meeks and colleagues[38] noted a significant difference in recurrence distal strictures between men with LS and those without LS (recurrence in LS 20.5%; no LS 7.5%; $P<.05$).

Treatment of pendulous stricture disease is driven by the quality of existent tissue and prior interventions. A one-stage repair with nongenital tissue, such as buccal mucosa, is feasible. However, various reports demonstrate a high failure rate with this approach.[35,39,40]

TWO-STAGE REPAIR

Extensive cases of urethral stricture disease due to LS with an inadequate native urethral plate for primary one-stage repair represent a reconstructive challenge. In these cases, a staged surgical approach often yields better outcomes than single-stage reconstruction.[41]

The first stage of this approach, as described by Barbagli, through a midline penile incision, involves complete excision of all affected urethra and full opening of the glans. Buccal mucosa is harvested and grafted to the tunica albuginea allowing for maturation over a 6- to 12-month

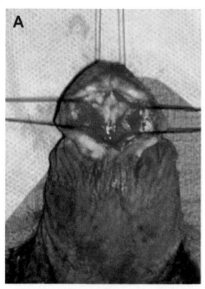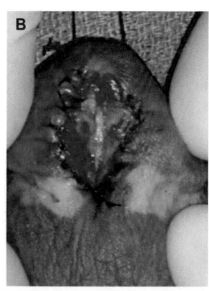

Fig. 6. (*A*) Meatotomy with exposed urethral plate and (*B*) Meatoplasty in patients with severe distal urethral stricture secondary to LS.

period. After the maturation process is complete, the graft is evaluated for appropriate take and recurrent LS. If the graft take is not acceptable or LS has recurred, then repeating the first stage may be required (**Fig. 7**). However, if the graft take is acceptable and free of recurrence, then one can proceed to the second stage. In these repairs, the use of fasciocutaneous flaps with genital skin is avoided secondary to disease recurrence in the genital skin.[37]

During the second stage, an approximately 28-mm-wide urethral plate is needed. This plate is incised and tubularized. Fistula formation is a known complication in patients with urethral stricture disease secondary to LS undergoing urethral reconstruction, with an incidence of approximately 1.9%.[39,42] To reduce fistula formation, closure with multiple layers in a nonoverlapping suture line technique and placement of a dartos or tunica vaginalis flap is recommended. The penile skin is then closed in the midline (**Fig. 8**).[41]

RECURRENCE AFTER 2-STAGE REPAIRS

The success rates for 2-stage repairs are traditionally lower when compared with uncomplicated urethral reconstruction, due to a variety of factors, including the extensive nature of preoperative urethral stricture disease and the recurrent nature of LS. Kulkarni and colleagues[43] demonstrated a recurrence rate of 27% at a mean follow-up time of 43 months for 2-stage buccal urethral reconstruction.

Peterson and colleagues[44] reported a series of 63 patients with LS, 19 who underwent first-stage repair. In this cohort, 11 patients ultimately underwent the second-stage reconstruction. They reported a recurrence rate of stricture in 2/11 (18%). Patel and colleagues[40] recently reported their observations in the management of stricture disease in patients with LS. Their cohort included

Fig. 7. Recurrence of LS after urethroplasty with buccal graft.

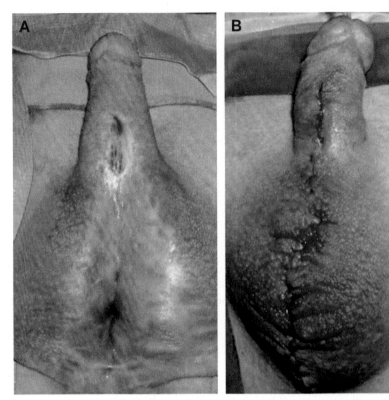

Fig. 8. (*A*) Healed first-stage urethroplasty. (*B*) Completed second-stage repair.

37 patients undergoing a 2-staged repair. Recurrence of LS was noted to occur on the first stage in 24% of the patients. Of the patients who underwent the second stage of their repair, recurrence was noted in 21% of those patients. These reports highlight the difficult challenge that LS poses on urethral reconstruction.

PERINEAL URETHROSTOMY

Perineal urethrostomy (PU) is a recognized alternative for proximal diversion in the nonsalvageable urethra. PU as the final point in management of an obstructed lower urinary tract is becoming more acceptable in men with LS and is an attractive option for patients with extensive urethral LS who may be unwilling or medically unfit to proceed with a 2-stage repair. Prior reports suggest patient satisfaction with a PU is acceptable.[41,44] Barbagli and colleagues[45] recently reported their experience in men undergoing PU demonstrating a 97% patient satisfaction rate.

The 2 main techniques, the Blandy PU and the "7-flap," use a wide-based perineal skin flap to avoid restenosis. In both cases, restenosis of the PU is minimized by the utilization of a flap instead of a puncture. The Blandy PU uses a posteriorly based skin flap raised through a U-shaped

perineal incision.[44] The proximal bulbar urethra is secured to the flap of perineal tissue with interrupted, absorbable sutures and matured at the skin level. Urinary continence is maintained because dissection is distal to the external urethral sphincter. The "7-flap," as described by French and colleagues,[46] uses a laterally based perineal skin flap. This flap is secured to the lateral aspect of the calibrated proximal bulbar urethral stump and matured at the skin level.

RECURRENCE WITH PERINEAL URETHROSTOMY

There is a wide range of reported recurrence for PU (72%–100%).[43,44] In his series of 173 patients, Barbagli reports a 70% success rate. Even though some patients needed up to 5 additional procedures, nearly all (97%) were satisfied with PU and would choose it again.[45] Peterson and colleagues[44] found that almost half of planned 2-stage repairs (8/19, 42%) elected to not proceed to the second stage, rendering them with a functional PU without significantly affecting quality of life.

Morey and colleagues[46] report a 90% success rate when using the "7-flap technique." Among those who failed, only endoscopic dilation was required, with no further open surgical revision needed. Patel and colleagues[40] also reported PU outcomes as a primary procedure of extensive urethral stricture disease. They noted a 93% success rate at a mean follow-up time of 14 months.

SUMMARY

LS is a progressive disease with a varied presentation and can be a challenging problem to manage. Localized disease to the foreskin and glans can be treated with potent topical steroids or circumcision. Urethral involvement occurs in 20% of patients. The extent of urethral involvement ranges from meatal only to panurethral. Intraurethral steroids with self-calibration may provide symptomatic relief to a large proportion of patients. Urethroplasty in this population has a higher risk of recurrence or need for multistage repairs to achieve a patent urethra. Last, in a highly selected group of patients, a PU may be advisable.

REFERENCES

1. New nomenclature for vulvar disease. Obstet Gynecol 1976;47(1):122–4.
2. Powell JJ, Wojnarowska F. Lichen sclerosus. Lancet 1999;353(9166):1777–83.
3. Das S, Tunuguntla HS. Balanitis xerotica obliterans–a review. World J Urol 2000;18(6):382–7.
4. Pugliese JM, Morey AF, Peterson AC. Lichen sclerosus: review of the literature and current recommendations for management. J Urol 2007;178(6):2268–76.
5. Riddell L, Edwards A, Sherrard J. Clinical features of lichen sclerosus in men attending a department of genitourinary medicine. Sex Transm Infect 2000; 76(4):311–3.
6. Azurdia RM, Luzzi GA, Byren I, et al. Lichen sclerosus in adult men: a study of HLA associations and susceptibility to autoimmune disease. Br J Dermatol 1999;140(1):79–83.
7. Laymon CW. Lichen sclerosus et atrophicus and related disorders. AMA Arch Derm Syphilol 1951; 64(5):620–7.
8. Regauer S. Immune dysregulation in lichen sclerosus. Eur J Cell Biol 2005;84(2–3):273–7.
9. Oyama N, Chan I, Neill SM, et al. Autoantibodies to extracellular matrix protein 1 in lichen sclerosus. Lancet 2003;362(9378):118–23.
10. Bjekic M, Sipetic S, Marinkovic J. Risk factors for genital lichen sclerosus in men. Br J Dermatol 2011;164(2):325–9.
11. Cantwell AR Jr. Histologic observations of pleomorphic, variably acid-fast bacteria in scleroderma, morphea, and lichen sclerosus et atrophicus. Int J Dermatol 1984;23(1):45–52.
12. Eisendle K, Grabner T, Kutzner H, et al. Possible role of Borrelia burgdorferi sensu lato infection in lichen sclerosus. Arch Dermatol 2008;144(5):591–8.
13. Farrell AM, Millard PR, Schomberg KH, et al. An infective aetiology for vulval lichen sclerosus re-addressed. Clin Exp Dermatol 1999;24(6):479–83.
14. Edmonds E, Mavin S, Francis N, et al. Borrelia burgdorferi is not associated with genital lichen sclerosus in men. Br J Dermatol 2009;160(2):459–60.
15. Pock L. Koebner phenomenon in lichen sclerosus et atrophicus. Dermatologica 1990;181(1):76–7.
16. Milligan A, Graham-Brown RA, Burns DA. Lichen sclerosus et atrophicus following sunburn. Clin Exp Dermatol 1988;13(1):36–7.
17. Yates VM, King CM, Dave VK. Lichen sclerosus et atrophicus following radiation therapy. Arch Dermatol 1985;121(8):1044–7.
18. Depasquale I, Park AJ, Bracka A. The treatment of balanitis xerotica obliterans. BJU Int 2000;86(4):459–65.
19. Barbagli G, Palminteri E, Mirri F, et al. Penile carcinoma in patients with genital lichen sclerosus: a multicenter survey. J Urol 2006;175(4):1359–63.
20. Powell J, Robson A, Cranston D, et al. High incidence of lichen sclerosus in patients with squamous cell carcinoma of the penis. Br J Dermatol 2001; 145(1):85–9.
21. Velazquez EF, Cubilla AL. Lichen sclerosus in 68 patients with squamous cell carcinoma of the penis: frequent atypias and correlation with special carcinoma variants suggests a precancerous role. Am J Surg Pathol 2003;27(11):1448–53.
22. Zaid UB, Lavien G, Potts B, et al. Malignancy in biopsy proven penile lichen sclerosus [abstract]. Munich (Germany): European Urology Association; 2016.
23. Meuli M, Briner J, Hanimann B, et al. Lichen sclerosus et atrophicus causing phimosis in boys: a prospective study with 5-year followup after complete circumcision. J Urol 1994;152(3):987–9.
24. Kiss A, Kiraly L, Kutasy B, et al. High incidence of balanitis xerotica obliterans in boys with phimosis: prospective 10-year study. Pediatr Dermatol 2005; 22(4):305–8.
25. Yardley IE, Cosgrove C, Lambert AW. Paediatric preputial pathology: are we circumcising enough? Ann R Coll Surg Engl 2007;89(1):62–5.
26. Wallace HJ. Lichen sclerosus et atrophicus. Trans St Johns Hosp Dermatol Soc 1971;57(1):9–30.
27. Kizer WS, Prarie T, Morey AF. Balanitis xerotica obliterans: epidemiologic distribution in an equal access health care system. South Med J 2003;96(1):9–11.
28. Nelson DM, Peterson AC. Lichen sclerosus: epidemiological distribution in an equal access health care system. J Urol 2011;185(2):522–5.
29. Liu JS, Walker K, Stein D, et al. Lichen sclerosus and isolated bulbar urethral stricture disease. J Urol 2014;192(3):775–9.

30. Palminteri E, Berdondini E, Verze P, et al. Contemporary urethral stricture characteristics in the developed world. Urology 2013;81(1):191–6.

31. Barbagli G, Palminteri E, Balo S, et al. Lichen sclerosus of the male genitalia and urethral stricture diseases. Urol Int 2004;73(1):1–5.

32. Belsante MJ, Selph JP, Peterson AC. The contemporary management of urethral strictures in men resulting from lichen sclerosus. Transl Androl Urol 2015;4(1):22–8.

33. Potts BA, Belsante MJ, Peterson AC. Intraurethral steroids are a safe and effective treatment for stricture disease in patients with biopsy-proven lichen sclerosus. J Urol 2016;195(6):1790–6.

34. Kyriakou A, Patsialas C, Patsatsi A, et al. Treatment of male genital lichen sclerosus with clobetasol propionate and maintenance with either methylprednisolone aceponate or tacrolimus: a retrospective study. J Dermatolog Treat 2013;24(6):431–4.

35. Tausch TJ, Peterson AC. Early aggressive treatment of lichen sclerosus may prevent disease progression. J Urol 2012;187(6):2101–5.

36. Morey AF, Lin HC, DeRosa CA, et al. Fossa navicularis reconstruction: impact of stricture length on outcomes and assessment of extended meatotomy (first stage Johanson) maneuver. J Urol 2007; 177(1):184–7 [discussion: 187].

37. Venn SN, Mundy AR. Urethroplasty for balanitis xerotica obliterans. Br J Urol 1998;81(5):735–7.

38. Meeks JJ, Barbagli G, Mehdiratta N, et al. Distal urethroplasty for isolated fossa navicularis and meatal strictures. BJU Int 2012;109(4):616–9.

39. Levine LA, Strom KH, Lux MM. Buccal mucosa graft urethroplasty for anterior urethral stricture repair: evaluation of the impact of stricture location and lichen sclerosus on surgical outcome. J Urol 2007; 178(5):2011–5.

40. Patel CK, Buckley JC, Zinman LN, et al. Outcomes for management of lichen sclerosus urethral strictures by 3 different techniques. Urology 2016;91: 215–21.

41. Barbagli G. When and how to use buccal mucosa grafts in penile and bulbar urethroplasty. Minerva Urol Nefrol 2004;56(2):189–203.

42. Acimovic M, Milojevic B, Milosavljevic M, et al. Primary dorsal buccal mucosa graft urethroplasty for anterior urethral strictures in patients with lichen sclerosus. Int Urol Nephrol 2016;48(4):541–5.

43. Kulkarni S, Barbagli G, Kirpekar D, et al. Lichen sclerosus of the male genitalia and urethra: surgical options and results in a multicenter international experience with 215 patients. Eur Urol 2009;55(4): 945–54.

44. Peterson AC, Palminteri E, Lazzeri M, et al. Heroic measures may not always be justified in extensive urethral stricture due to lichen sclerosus (balanitis xerotica obliterans). Urology 2004;64(3):565–8.

45. Barbagli G, De Angelis M, Romano G, et al. Clinical outcome and quality of life assessment in patients treated with perineal urethrostomy for anterior urethral stricture disease. J Urol 2009;182(2):548–57.

46. French D, Hudak SJ, Morey AF. The "7-flap" perineal urethrostomy. Urology 2011;77(6):1487–9.

Treatment of Radiation-Induced Urethral Strictures

Matthias D. Hofer, MD[a], Joceline S. Liu, MD[b],
Allen F. Morey, MD[a],*

KEYWORDS

- Urethroplasty • Prostate cancer • Radiation therapy

KEY POINTS

- Most radiation-induced urethral strictures occur in the bulbomembranous junction, and urinary incontinence may result as a consequence of treatment.
- Radiation therapy may compromise reconstruction due to poor tissue healing and radionecrosis.
- Excision and primary anastomosis is the preferred urethroplasty technique for radiation-induced urethral stricture.
- Principles of posterior urethroplasty for trauma may be applied to the treatment of radiation-induced urethral strictures.
- Chronic management with suprapubic tube is an option based on patient comorbidities and preference.

RADIATION THERAPY AND URETHRAL STRICTURES

Prostate cancer remains the most common cancer in men with more than 200,000 new cases anticipated each year.[1] Common management options for prostate cancer include surgery, in the form of radical prostatectomy, or radiation therapy with external beam radiation (EBR), brachytherapy (BT), or a combination of both therapies.[2] Jarosek and colleagues noted that most patients (about 70%) elect radiotherapy compared with about 30% choosing surgery.[3]

Urethral strictures have been reported to occur in 2% of patients undergoing EBR, 4% to 32% for BT therapy depending on the dose, and 11% of EBR-BT combination therapy.[4,5] Risk factors

for the development of radiation-induced strictures include transurethral resection of the prostate before radiation, regardless of whether EBR or BT was used,[6] as well as age, non-white race, low income, and increased comorbidity status (BT use only).[7] Ionizing radiation leads to direct tissue damage in the form of DNA damage and indirect damage via free radical formation within cells—both resulting in cellular apoptosis and subsequent replacement of functional tissue with scar. An additional consequence of radiation therapy contributing to the development of urethral strictures is vascular damage in the form of obliterative endarteritis.[8]

Analysis of trends in treatment over the last decade suggests that radiation therapy continues to grow in popularity for the treatment of both

Disclosure: None of the authors have any involvement, financial or otherwise, to disclose that might potentially pose conflict of interest.
[a] Department of Urology, University of Texas Southwestern, Dallas, TX, USA; [b] Department of Urology, Feinberg School of Medicine, Northwestern University, Chicago, IL, USA
* Corresponding author. 5323 Harry Hines Boulevard, Dallas, TX 75390-9110.
E-mail address: allen.morey@utsouthwestern.edu

clinically localized and locally advanced prostate cancer.[9,10] This rising utilization trend, along with the characteristic lag-time from radiation exposure to clinically significant urethral stricture of more than 6 years,[11] contributes to what is expected will be an increase in patients presenting with radiation-induced urethral strictures.

THE CHALLENGE OF TREATING RADIATION-INDUCED URETHRAL STRICTURES

Several factors complicate repair of radiation-induced urethral strictures:

- Most of these strictures are located in the bulbomembranous urethra, which is a challenging position for repair because of difficulty in access. This location also confers the danger of rendering the patient incontinent after the procedure if the sphincter is involved in or damaged during the stricture repair or by radiation fibrosis itself.
- The commonly encountered radionecrosis of the prostate (**Fig. 1**) further impedes performing urethral anastomosis because sutures tend to tear through the necrotic tissue unless they are completely removed.
- The poor vascularity of the radiated tissue also impedes the healing process after urethroplasty,[12] contributing to the high recurrence rate following urethral stricture treatment compared with posttraumatic repairs. Recurrence rates are reported as high as 30%[11,13] in radiation-induced strictures repair compared with about 16% recurrence rate of urethral strictures overall.

Accurate diagnosis of the nature of the stricture is strongly recommended. A combined examination with a retrograde urethrogram (RUG) and voiding cystourethrogram (VCUG) is ideal to delineate features such as the location, length, and severity of the stricture (**Fig. 2**). This examination subsequently allows the surgeon to plan the surgical approach—perineal versus abdominoperineal, with or without pubectomy. The authors believe that one critical concept in the treatment of radiation-induced urethral strictures is urethral rest,[14] allowing for the stricture to declare itself in the fullest extent. Cystoscopy at the time of suprapubic tube placement may be a useful addition to the diagnostic workup, specifically to gauge the amount of radionecrosis. Further imaging with computed tomography or MRI is rarely beneficial in further delineating the stricture, but may be useful in cases of assessing neighboring organs for abnormality or those with concomitant fistula. Sexual function including erectile and ejaculatory competence should be recorded before surgical management of urethral strictures and reassessed postoperatively. Baseline erectile function may be preserved in 50% of patients undergoing urethroplasty procedures after radiation therapy, whereas ejaculatory function has not been studied in this setting.[11]

SURGICAL MANAGEMENT APPROACHES
Endoscopic Management

Endoscopic management including dilation and direct visual internal urethrotomy (DVIU) of radiation-induced strictures as first-line treatment has been proposed,[15] but should be discouraged especially after repeat recurrences. The risk of recurrence is reportedly nearly 50% in patients who underwent BT,[7] but the true incidence of recurrence is likely much higher. In addition, repeated urethral dilations and DVIU attempts often cause further fibrosis of irradiated tissues along with treatment delays.

The UroLume Approach

Over the course of the last 40 years, the treatment armamentarium to these strictures has evolved.

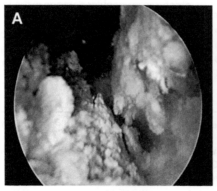
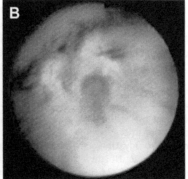

Fig. 1. Examples of cystoscopic images of radiation-induced urethral strictures. (*A*) Extensive radionecrosis of the prostate. (*B*) Complete urethral obliteration.

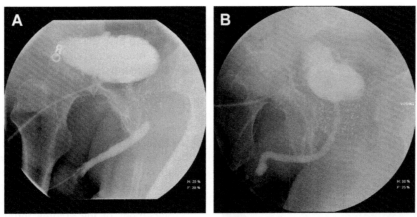

Fig. 2. Preoperative and postoperative images of the same patient. (*A*) RUG and VCUG show an approximately 6-cm obliterated stricture of the prostatic and membranous urethra in this patient after BT. (*B*) Postoperative VCUG demonstrates a patent urethra.

Initial studies after the introduction of the UroLume urethral stent were promising, reporting success rates reaching 85% at 20 months of follow-up.[7,16,17] Accordingly, the UroLume (American Medical Systems, Minnetonka, MN) stent became applied as a minimally invasive, endoscopic treatment option for radiation-induced strictures for those not in favor of open surgery.[16] The maintenance of urethral patency with the UroLume was often associated with sphincter damage resulting in incontinence in up to 96% of men.[16] However, with extended follow-up, the initial enthusiasm for UroLume stents began to wane as its role was called into question.[18] UroLume patients often required at least 2 additional endoscopic procedures for stent-related obstruction, including stent migration, ingrowth, or calcification.[18]

Given the high complication and stent failure rate, the UroLume was removed from the US market in 2013. Although UroLume stent placement thereafter has become obsolete, sequelae and complications related to the stent may continue to present for many years. One of the consequences of the Uro-Lume is the ingrowth of urethral tissue and incorporation of the stent into the urethral wall, making subsequent re-treatment or definitive excision and reconstruction nearly impossible. In the authors' experience, the many men failing initial UroLume stents for treatment of radiation-induced stricture recurrences required eventual urinary diversion due to complete destruction of the urethra.

Perineal Surgery: Excision and Primary Anastomosis

The authors believe that excision and primary anastomosis (EPA) is a superior approach for the treatment of radiation-induced urethral strictures. They perform the following steps:

- Urethral rest before surgery is advised.[14] The authors achieve this with initial cystourethroscopy and placement of a suprapubic tube, left in place 2 to 3 months before reconstruction is attempted. Urethral rest allows for the stricture to declare itself fully and it also decreases periurethral inflammation, which impedes both dissection of the urethra and removal of scar tissue and may also impede wound healing following urethroplasty. The authors treat symptomatic bacteriuria before surgery, and asymptomatic bacteriuria with intraoperative coverage with intravenous broad-spectrum antibiotics.

- The authors perform EPA through a midline perineal incision in high lithotomy position using a Lone Star Retractor for exposure. In case of narrow strictures (**Fig. 3**) or if the patient does not have a suprapubic tube allowing for antegrade access, they place a wire through the stricture cystoscopically to aid in identification of the true lumen because the often densely scarred corpus spongiosum can obscure it.

- Once the dissection through the perineal fat is completed and the bulbospongiosus muscle is divided, the urethra is mobilized. Once freed from the perineal body as much as tentatively necessary based on the preoperative imaging results, the exact location is defined with cystoscopy and the urethra is transected. The authors attempt to transect through the stricture rather than distal to it. They first remove urethral and spongiosal scar tissue from the distal end followed by spatulation to allow for a 24-French calibration with a bougie à boule. They then mobilize the distal stump of the urethra aggressively, freeing it

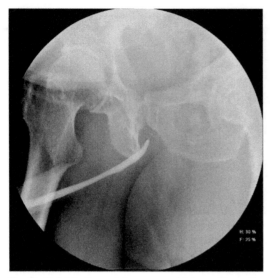

Fig. 3. Tight bulbomembraneous stricture. Here, the authors recommend placing a guidewire cystoscopically at the beginning of the operation to aid in the identification of the urethral lumen when resecting scar tissue.

from its attachment to the corpora and from periurethral tissue.

- The next (and most critical) step is resection of the scar of the proximal aspect of the urethra. Here, it is important to remove all urethral scar tissue in its entirety as otherwise a stricture recurrence is likely. This removal of all urethral scar tissue often can be best performed using a number 15 blade, but the authors have found that the use of a rongeur is very helpful for this maneuver. A wire placed at the beginning of the procedure is a useful guide to maintain control of the proximal urethral lumen when suprapubic access does not exist.

- In cases in which the stricture has rendered the urethral lumen completely obliterated, the authors insert an 18-French van Buren sound through the suprapubic cystostomy tract and through the bladder neck. This maneuver allows the delineation of the proximal (patent) aspect of the urethra visually and by palpation. The authors place traction sutures (4-0 Vicryl) at the lateral aspects of the scar tissue that they presume to be the proximal urethral stump containing the obliterated lumen. They then use the number 15 blade scalpel to cut in the midline of the scar onto the tip of the sound between the traction sutures until they reach the proximal lumen. Scar tissue being held up by the traction sutures can now easily be removed.

- Next, the authors thoroughly inspect the prostate, because all necrotic tissue will have to be removed. It is impossible to place proximal anastomotic sutures in necrotic tissue, because they will tear through and/or a stricture recurrence will develop. The authors recommend the removal of any remaining periurethral scar tissue, which may involve the periosteum of the symphysis pubis. Again, the use of a rongeur has been proven to be very useful.

- Once all scar and necrotic prostate tissue have been removed, the authors place 12 absorbable sutures of 5-0 polydioxanone (PDS) through the proximal urethral stump. Using double-armed needles allows for easier placement of the sutures through the right aspect of the urethra because they can be placed forehand and inside out, leaving one needle on the inside of the lumen after cutting the suture in half. The remaining single-armed suture can now be placed outside-to-in on the left aspect of the urethra, again leaving the needle at the inside position.

- The authors routinely perform a cystoscopic evaluation of the bladder at this point, especially if the patient has had a suprapubic tube for an extended period of time. Bladder stones are removed if encountered.

- The authors next place their anastomotic sutures through the distal stump of the urethra in a counterclockwise fashion starting at 12 o'clock. As all needles are on the inside of the lumen of the proximal stump, they can easily place them inside out in the distal urethral stump. Care is taken to insert a 14-French silicone catheter once half of the sutures have been placed to avoid entangling of the catheter when the knots are tied at the end of this step.

- The authors attempt to place a second suture layer with running 5-0 PDS in the form of a spongioplasty, although often there is insufficient spongiosal tissue on the proximal aspect.

- Last, the authors close the incision with 2 layers of running 2-0 Monocryl and the skin with interrupted 3-0 chromic sutures. The authors do not routinely leave a drain. Application of hemostatic agents such as oxidized regenerated cellulose may be indicated. Antibiotic coverage is maintained with a prophylactic dose of a macrobid antibiotic for the duration of catheterization. They perform a VCUG at 3 weeks and remove the catheter if no contrast extravasation is seen.

Successful and durable reconstruction can be achieved in nearly three-quarters of patients.[11]

The authors have recently found that with increasing experience success rates are as high as 85% with a 2-year follow-up. Late recurrences are rare (2.7%). Incontinence can occur in 7% to 19% of patients[11,19] as the tradeoff for the necessary scar removal involving the membranous urethra. Staged placement of an artificial urinary sphincter, however, is a suitable treatment for these men.[11] Sexual function in patients after EPA appears to be unchanged, and rates of postoperative erectile dysfunction are consistent with previously reported rates in the postradiation setting.[20]

Abdominoperineal Anastomosis

In rare cases, the stricture is located so proximally that a perineal approach alone is insufficient to complete scar excision and reanastomosis of the urethra to the bladder neck or proximal urethral stump. In this case, the authors proceed with a perineal dissection as outlined earlier. In addition, they perform a midline abdominal incision to mobilize the bladder, because this is the necessary step to gain sufficient length for an anastomosis. The authors are often able to connect with the perineal dissection lateral or anterior to the proximal urethral stump. The dorsal venous plexus in irradiated patients is obliterated and does not constitute an obstacle. At this point, it has proven to be useful to open the bladder in the vertical midline between stay sutures to insert an 18-French bougie à boule in antegrade fashion. This maneuver allows delineating the rendezvous point with the perineal dissection of the distal stump. In some instances, the pubic bone is overlying the site of the anastomosis prohibiting sufficient exposure. Here, the authors use osteotomes to remove part of the pubic bone, most commonly at the inferior aspect. Usually, removal of a 2- to 3-cm fragment is sufficient and the pelvic stability is not impaired. The anastomosis is now performed in identical fashion to the perineal approach.

Urethroplasty Using Grafts or Flaps

Although urethroplasty with grafts and flaps has been reported with success rates of 71% to 83%,[11,19] the authors prefer the EPA technique, because transfer of tissue such as buccal mucosa grafts into an irradiated recipient area with poor vascularity due to radiation-induced damage is unlikely to succeed. Similarly, genital fasciocutaneous flaps in an irradiated patient are often unwieldly.[21] If tissue transfer is necessary, the combination of buccal mucosa grafts and gracilis muscle flaps is possible.[22] The gracilis muscle provides a vascular bed for ventral onlay of a buccal mucosal graft, which otherwise would not be able to develop sufficient neovascularization. A success rate of this procedure of 78% in the irradiated patient has been reported.[22]

Management with Chronic Suprapubic Tube

Urinary diversion in the management of the irradiated patient serves a dual purpose—that of urethral rest and as long-term management in the properly counseled patient. As previously stated, the authors found that urethral rest allows tissue recovery, without need for urethral catheterization or manipulation, and facilitates more accurate declaration of stricture severity and involvement as an aid to surgical planning.[14] The importance of complete excision of necrotic or fibrotic tissue at the time of reconstruction cannot be overemphasized. At the authors' institution, all patients will undergo a period of 2 to 3 months of urethral rest with suprapubic drainage before reconstruction. Following this period of urinary drainage, patients may either choose to proceed to surgical reconstruction or elect to continue with chronic suprapubic tube drainage. Chronic suprapubic tube remains an option in cases when surgery is not advisable from a medical standpoint. Some patients may also prefer to avoid surgery in favor of drainage, because it often significantly improves incontinence. In the authors' experience, almost half (45.6%) of patients presenting for consultation elected to continue with chronic suprapubic tube drainage rather than proceeding to reconstruction.

SUMMARY

Management of radiation-induced urethral strictures is challenging, and the authors expect the number of patients presenting with these strictures to increase. The recommended treatment is a surgical urethral reconstruction with EPA, which shows durable success in the vast majority of patients.

REFERENCES

1. Mohler JL, Kantoff PW, Armstrong AJ, et al. Prostate cancer, version 2.2014. J Natl Compr Canc Netw 2014;12:686–718.
2. Thompson I, Thrasher JB, Aus G, et al. Guideline for the management of clinically localized prostate cancer: 2007 update. J Urol 2007;177:2106–31.
3. Jarosek SL, Virnig BA, Chu H, et al. Propensity-weighted long-term risk of urinary adverse events after prostate cancer surgery, radiation, or both. Eur Urol 2015;67(2):273–80.
4. Mohammed N, Kestin L, Ghilezan M, et al. Comparison of acute and late toxicities for three modern high-dose radiation treatment techniques for

localized prostate cancer. Int J Radiat Oncol Biol Phys 2012;82:204–12.

5. Hindson BR, Millar JL, Matheson B. Urethral strictures following high-dose-rate brachytherapy for prostate cancer: analysis of risk factors. Brachytherapy 2013;12:50–5.

6. Gardner BG, Zietman AL, Shipley WU, et al. Late normal tissue sequelae in the second decade after high dose radiation therapy with combined photons and conformal protons for locally advanced prostate cancer. J Urol 2002;167:123–6.

7. Sullivan L, Williams SG, Tai KH, et al. Urethral stricture following high dose rate brachytherapy for prostate cancer. Radiother Oncol 2009;91:232–6.

8. Tibbs MK. Wound healing following radiation therapy: a review. Radiother Oncol 1997;42:99–106.

9. Cooperberg MR, Broering JM, Carroll PR. Time trends and local variation in primary treatment of localized prostate cancer. J Clin Oncol 2010;28:1117–23.

10. Cooperberg MR, Carroll PR. Trends in management for patients with localized prostate cancer, 1990-2013. JAMA 2015;314:80–2.

11. Hofer MD, Zhao LC, Morey AF, et al. Outcomes after urethroplasty for radiotherapy induced bulbomembranous urethral stricture disease. J Urol 2014;191:1307–12.

12. Elliott SP, Meng MV, Elkin EP, et al. Incidence of urethral stricture after primary treatment for prostate cancer: data From CaPSURE. J Urol 2007;178:529–34 [discussion: 34].

13. Elliott SP, McAninch JW, Chi T, et al. Management of severe urethral complications of prostate cancer therapy. J Urol 2006;176:2508–13.

14. Terlecki RP, Steele MC, Valadez C, et al. Urethral rest: role and rationale in preparation for anterior urethroplasty. Urology 2011;77:1477–81.

15. Herschorn S, Elliott S, Coburn M, et al. SIU/ICUD consultation on urethral strictures: posterior urethral stenosis after treatment of prostate cancer. Urology 2014;83:S59–70.

16. Erickson BA, McAninch JW, Eisenberg ML, et al. Management for prostate cancer treatment related posterior urethral and bladder neck stenosis with stents. J Urol 2011;185:198–203.

17. Eisenberg ML, Elliott SP, McAninch JW. Preservation of lower urinary tract function in posterior urethral stenosis: selection of appropriate patients for urethral stents. J Urol 2007;178:2456–60 [discussion: 60–1].

18. McNamara ER, Webster GD, Peterson AC. The UroLume stent revisited: the Duke experience. Urology 2013;82:933–6.

19. Glass AS, McAninch JW, Zaid UB, et al. Urethroplasty after radiation therapy for prostate cancer. Urology 2012;79:1402–5.

20. Beard CJ, Propert KJ, Rieker PP, et al. Complications after treatment with external-beam irradiation in early-stage prostate cancer patients: a prospective multiinstitutional outcomes study. J Clin Oncol 1997;15:223–9.

21. Meeks JJ, Brandes SB, Morey AF, et al. Urethroplasty for radiotherapy induced bulbomembranous strictures: a multi-institutional experience. J Urol 2011;185:1761–5.

22. Palmer DA, Buckley JC, Zinman LN, et al. Urethroplasty for high-risk, long segment urethral strictures with ventral buccal mucosa graft and gracilis muscle flap. J Urol 2014;193(3):902–5.

Urethral Strictures and Artificial Urinary Sphincter Placement

Jeremy B. Myers, MD*, William O. Brant, MD,
James N. Hotaling, MD, MS, Sara M. Lenherr, MD, MS

KEYWORDS

- Artificial urinary sphincter • Urethral stricture • Incontinence • Erosion • Complication

KEY POINTS

- Patients undergoing artificial urinary sphincter (AUS) placement often have complex medical and surgical histories, such as radical prostatectomy, endoscopic treatment of urethral strictures, previous AUS placement, and prior open urethral surgery.
- Urethral strictures at the bladder neck, membranous urethra, or site of a previous AUS erosion are problems that profoundly affect the timing and treatment success of AUS placement.
- Understanding the complexities and outcomes in this subset of patients is the only way to inform shared decision making about treatment of urinary incontinence.

BACKGROUND

The artificial urinary sphincter (AUS) was pioneered by Dr F. Brantley Scott in collaboration with University of Minnesota and was first implanted in approximately 1972. There are several AUSs available; however, the most commonly used by far is the AMS 800 (American Medical Systems, Minnetonka, MN). The AMS 800 has been available since 1987 after introduction of a narrow-backed urethral cuff (acting to more safely distribute pressure to the urethra). Other modifications have included a quick-connect tubing system, antibiotic coating, and smaller cuff sizes. However, the essential design of the current AMS 800 has undergone little change in the last 30 years.

The AUS is irrefutably the gold standard for treatment of high-volume postprostatectomy incontinence and it is estimated that it has been implanted in more than 150,000 patients worldwide.[1] In a 2013 systematic review, continence rates (defined as $\leq$1 pad per day) vary from 61% to 100% after AUS implantation.[1] Patient satisfaction was also high and in the few studies the few studies that reported various measures of quality of life (QoL), including the American Urologic Association QoL index and the Incontinence Impact Questionnaire Short Form, showed significant improvements after AUS implantation.[1] The trade-off for this improved QoL in patients after AUS placement is a high revision rate. These revisions arise from a variety of causes, such as lack of initial efficacy, urethral atrophy, erosion, infection, and mechanical failure. Some studies report as high as 53% revision rate in the first 5 years after implantation even at tertiary referral centers.[2]

The complexity of surgical care for patients undergoing AUS placement is highlighted by the procedures surgical learning curve.[3] Patients needing

Disclosures: Dr W.O. Brant is a paid proctor, consultant, and investigator for Boston Scientific. Dr W.O. Brant is on the safety advisory board of GT Urologic. Drs W.O. Brant and J.B. Myers coadminister a reconstructive urologic fellowship, which receives educational support from Boston Scientific.
Genitourinary Injury and Reconstructive Urology, Department of Surgery, University of Utah, 30 North 1900 East, Room # 3B420, Salt Lake City, UT 84132, USA
* Corresponding author.
E-mail address: Jeremy.myers@hsc.utah.edu

urologic.theclinics.com

AUS implantation often a have past history of pelvic irradiation, AUS erosion, rectourethral fistula, prior urethroplasty, and urethral stricture or bladder neck contracture. Describing outcomes for AUS placement in the setting of such complex anatomy is essential to counsel patients about their risks, and understand whether further revision surgery for urinary incontinence is in their best interests. This article reviews the recent evidence regarding urethral strictures/bladder neck contracture and how these conditions affect the use of AUS in incontinent men.

This article is divided view into 3 categories that pertain to different aspects of urethral stricture or bladder neck contracture and AUS placement. These categories are:

- Bladder neck contracture and AUS placement.
- Management of AUS erosion and subsequent stricture risk.
- AUS placement after urethral reconstruction or urethroplasty.

BLADDER NECK CONTRACTURE AND ARTIFICIAL URINARY SPHINCTER PLACEMENT
Incidence of Bladder Neck Contracture

Bladder neck contracture is a common occurrence after prostate surgery. The most common surgical causes are radical prostatectomy for prostate cancer and transurethral prostate surgery for benign prostatic enlargement (BPE). In a recent Surveillance Epidemiology and End Results (SEER)–Medicare analysis the cumulative incidence of bladder outlet obstruction after radical prostatectomy was 5% greater than that of controls and 12% higher for men who were also receiving adjuvant or salvage radiotherapy after radical prostatectomy.[4] These findings are similar to those of other large population-based studies of prostate cancer treatment complications, in which the cumulative need for either internal urethrotomy or incision of bladder neck contracture after radical prostatectomy was 7.5% to 8.4%.[5,6] The advent of robotic-assisted radical prostatectomy and the ability to perform continuous and precise suturing of the vesicourethral anastomosis has been shown in some single-center studies to decrease the rate of bladder neck contracture,[7,8] whereas in other studies this has not been shown to be true.[9,10]

Transurethral prostate surgeries for BPE also can result in bladder neck contracture. A recent meta-analysis of 31 trials comparing monopolar with bipolar transurethral resection of the prostate (TURP) reported a pooled 3.5% incidence of bladder neck contracture.[11] Incontinence after TURP is rare, but in some studies of AUS placement that reported on patients with mixed causes of incontinence, post-TURP incontinence was the reason for implant in 7.5% to 18.5% of cases.[2,12]

Endoscopic Management of Bladder Neck Contracture

The first-line treatment of bladder neck contracture, regardless of its cause, is generally endoscopic management. Some studies show that endoscopic management is successful in greater than 80% of bladder neck contractures with a single transurethral incision of the bladder neck (TUIBN).[13] A recent analysis of SEER-Medicare data for the burden of bladder outlet obstruction in men after treatment of prostate cancer showed at a median of 8.8 years that 56% of men required only 1 procedure for bladder neck contracture.[14] More recent studies have focused on recalcitrant bladder neck contractures that have not responded to initial endoscopic management, and the success of further endoscopic interventions before AUS placement. The Lahey Clinic published a recent small series of men undergoing treatment of bladder neck contracture with intralesional injection of mitomycin C at the time of TUIBN.[15] They found very high success (72%) at a median follow-up of 12 months with this approach despite most of the men having failed prior endoscopic management. The Trauma and Urologic Reconstruction Network of Surgeons (TURNS; TURNSresearch.org) subsequently published a retrospective case series of men undergoing treatment of bladder neck contracture with mitomycin C injection.[16] The study had major limitations because there were a variety of mitomycin C doses and endoscopic techniques. However, the strength of the study was a strict criterion for anatomic success based on cystoscopic examination. They found a lower success rate of 58% at a median follow-up of 9.2 months compared with the Lahey Clinic study; however, because of restricting follow-up to men with cystoscopic examination only, asymptomatic recurrences were detected, thus decreasing the overall apparent success. Other contemporary studies report similar or better outcomes to the TURNS study with endoscopic management alone (no injection). These studies vary by follow-up protocols and reporting of how many procedures were required, but the successful resolution of bladder neck contracture with endoscopic management was 72% to 73%.[17,18] These study results are summarized in **Table 1**. In all of these recent studies, investigators emphasize the need for a deep incision to perivesical fat with either a urethrotomy or Collins hot knife (**Fig. 1**). Some factors that influenced the success of the procedure were smoking and 2 or more previous failed endoscopic procedures.[18]

Table 1
Studies characterizing treatment of recalcitrant bladder neck contractures and subsequent treatment of incontinence with artificial urinary sphincter placement

Study	N	Follow-up (mo)	Prior Treatment BNCX (%)	Cause (%)	XRT (%)	BNCX Treatment Success	Incontinence	AUS Placements	AUS/BNCX Failures	Other Findings
Anger et al,[29] 2005	35 (nonobliterated BNCX)	Mean 22.6	43	RP: 100	15	1 procedure: 100%	100% preoperative	AUS 100% (94% placed at time of BNCX treatment)	AUS: 9 of 35 (26%) revision at mean 31 mo BNCX: no recurrences	—
Ramirez et al,[18] 2013	50	Mean 12.9	78	RP: 74 TURP: 26	4	1 procedure: 36 (72%) 2 procedures: 7 + 36 = 43 (86%)	78% preoperative, 80% postoperative	24 of 43 (56%) AUS at mean 2.9 mo	AUS: 5 of 24 (21%) no erosions BNCX: 2 recurrences at 5 and 7 mo	Predictors of BNCX treatment failure: smoking, ≥2 failed previous procedures
Brede C et al,[17] 2014	63	Median 11	100	RP: 100	27	Unspecified number of procedures 46 (73%)	—	33 of 46 (72%)	AUS: 2 of 33 (6%) 1 erosion BNCX: 0	—
Redshaw et al,[16] 2015	55	Median 9.2 (cystoscopic)	80	RP: 60 TURP: 22	25	1 procedure: 32 (53%) 2 procedures 9 + 21 = 41 (75%)	—	—	—	Median recurrence of BNCX 3.7 mo

Abbreviations: BNCX, bladder neck contracture; RP, radical prostatectomy; XRT, radiation therapy.

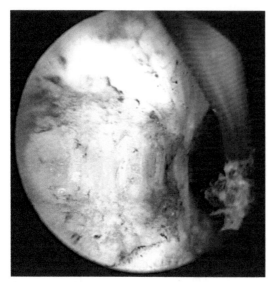

Fig. 1. Deep incisions up to the level of the capsule and or perivesical fat are essential to successful endoscopic resolution of bladder neck contracture.

A recent white paper released from the AUS consensus group, sponsored by the International Continence Society, suggested a balanced and reasonable treatment algorithm for bladder neck contracture before AUS placement.[19] The group suggested that men undergo standard TUIBN or dilation; if this fails they should have aggressive endoscopic management of the contracture. If endoscopic management fails to resolve the bladder neck contracture or there was complete urethral obliteration, then open urethral reconstruction should be performed.[19]

Another management strategy for bladder neck contracture before treatment of incontinence with AUS implantation is use of a urethral stent. The UroLume endoprosthesis or stent (American Medical Systems, Minnetonka, MN) was an expandable metal stent that was recently withdrawn from the market by AMS. The intention of the Uro-Lume was to expand to about 30 French and then epithelialize and incorporate into the wall of the urethra, serving as an alternative to urethroplasty. The initial results were promising for the treatment of urethral strictures, but longer-term experience revealed that patients often had worsening progressive stricture at either end of the UroLume, obstruction of the stent with fibrosis, and very poor patient satisfaction.[20,21] In addition, subsequent urethroplasty was significantly more complicated after UroLume placement.[22] The UroLume stent was also used for a variety of other indications, including the treatment of BPE, detrusor sphincter dyssynergia, and recalcitrant bladder neck contracture.

Several centers were proponents of treatment of recalcitrant bladder neck contracture with placement of the UroLume stent. Even though the Uro-Lume is off the market and there are currently no alternative urethral stents available in the United States, management of urethral strictures in the setting of a UroLume stent warrants discussion because there are still many patients with these in place. The University of California, San Francisco (UCSF) reported the use of the UroLume for treatment of posterior urethral stricture (including bladder neck contracture) in 2007, mostly in patients after radiation therapy for prostate cancer, and noted that although there was a high intervention rate for restenosis and stent obstruction, the stent only had to be removed in 15% of patients.[23] The ability to successfully manage posterior urethral restenosis was in contrast with stent obstruction in the anterior urethra, where the stents almost always had to be removed in a urethroplasty to prevent restenosis.[24] The investigators updated their series in 2010 and found that in 38 men with obstruction of the posterior urethra the success was only 47%, with the remaining 53% of men requiring 1.6 procedures each with only 2.3 years of average follow-up.[25] In an editorial in *Journal of Urology,* investigators from UCSF concluded that, "In our experience open surgical reconstruction is superior to UroLume stenting in patients with a reasonable life expectancy, and favorable cancer and health status."[26]

Other centers also reported a similar rate of resolution of bladder neck contracture and/or urethral stenosis after UroLume. Duke reported a 53% rate of resolution of stenosis at an average of 55 months of follow-up with the UroLume, but the investigators had to perform an average of 2.4 procedures in patients with restenosis or ingrowth of the urethral stent.[27] Mayo clinic reported almost exactly the same results in 25 men: 52% stabilization of bladder neck contracture after a first procedure at a median follow-up of 2.9 years.[28] Although this is largely a moot point because the UroLume stent is no longer available, the contemporary concerns associated with the UroLume are worsening of the stricture and inflammatory process, which can lead to chronic (in some cases debilitating) discomfort in the perineum, intractable irritative bladder symptoms, and inability to subsequently reconstruct the lower urinary tract after UroLume placement.

Incontinence Rates After Treatment of Bladder Neck Contracture

Incontinence rates can be very high after treatment of bladder neck contracture, especially in men after radical prostatectomy and in patients with recalcitrant contractures. First-time treatment of bladder neck contracture may not carry nearly as much risk of incontinence, with 83% of patients reporting no problems or very slight problems with urinary leakage.[13] Subsequent treatment of recurrent contractures has a much higher risk because the bladder neck contracture often occurs essentially within the membranous sphincter. It is paramount that patients are warned about this eventuality with treatment of the contracture. In recent reports on the treatment of recalcitrant contractures, the rate of AUS placement for incontinence varied and preoperative incontinence was often not quantified (see **Table 1**). There was a 56% to 100% rate of AUS placement in these studies. However, AUS placement as a proxy for postoperative incontinence probably underestimates the problem substantially because many men in whom TUIBN failed may still be incontinent (leaking essentially through a fixed strictured area). Because of recurrent contracture these incontinent men may not be candidates for AUS placement and thus the rates of overall incontinence in these studies may be even higher.

Placement of Artificial Urinary Sphincter After Endoscopic Treatment of Bladder Neck Contracture

Establishing the stability of the bladder neck or strictured area is essential before placement of an AUS, because, after AUS placement, further endoscopic management can be limited and lead to an AUS complication. How long to wait before placement of an AUS is not well understood. In some cases, bladder neck contractures can recur very slowly over time and most men do not tolerate prolonged waiting periods, such as a year, which would be required to safely identify all recurrences before treatment of their incontinence. The endoscopic appearance of the bladder neck after TUIBN and the surgeon's judgment about healing in the area is probably the best guide. Those contractures that occur without a history of pelvic irradiation and are well healed without contracture (**Fig. 2**) probably can have placement of an AUS at 3 months, whereas those patients with necrosis, poor healing, or a history of radiotherapy probably warrant a longer observation time.

Data supporting this approach are varied. For instance, investigators from Duke University advocated TUIBN and concomitant placement of an AUS.[29] At almost 2 years of follow-up, 100% of men had successful resolution and no reinterventions for stenosis. Although their cohort included only nonobliterated bladder neck contractures,

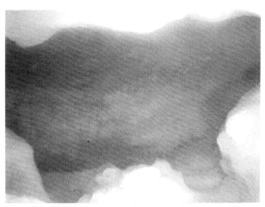

Fig. 2. Example of excellent healing after transurethral incision of bladder neck. Note the lateral incisions at the 4 and 8 o'clock positions.

they were nevertheless complex patients, with 43% having prior endoscopic treatment and 15% having previous radiotherapy. In contrast, in the TURNS study previously mentioned, the median time to recurrence was 3.7 months, and Kaplan-Meier analysis showed appreciable continued recurrence rates after this time.[16] In addition, the study reported a median follow-up of only 9 months and likely underestimated the ultimate recurrence rate. However, the TURNS cohort included a higher rate of previously failed treatment (80%) and history of pelvic radiotherapy (25%) compared with the Duke study.

Although there are limited data to guide surgeons, the authors advocate the individualized timing of AUS placement after management of bladder neck contracture. This timing should be guided by the endoscopic appearance of the bladder neck at 3 to 4 months after incision, previous history of radiotherapy, failed prior TUIBN, and smoking status.

MANAGEMENT OF ARTIFICIAL URINARY SPHINCTER EROSION AND SUBSEQUENT STRICTURE RISK
Risk of Artificial Urinary Sphincter Erosion

AUS erosion is a rare but serious complication for patients because of the ensuing infection that results from the erosion; the complexity of management of the damaged urethra, which can lead to stricture and fistulization to the perineum; and the protracted course until reimplantation of another AUS (if even possible). The rates of AUS erosion vary considerably depending on many patient factors. The largest single study, from the Mayo clinic, recently reported erosion in 6% of 497 patients undergoing first-time AUS placement at a median follow-up of 2 years.[30] Other studies report a range of erosion rates from 2% to 13% depending on patient characteristics.[2,30–34] Patient factors that have been associated with an increased risk of AUS erosion are coronary artery disease, hypertension, and prior pelvic radiotherapy. Surgical factors associated with AUS erosion are previous AUS revision surgery, prior AUS erosion, double cuff placement, UroLume stenting, prior urethroplasty, use of a 3.5-cm cuff, and placement of a urethral catheter by outside hospitals.[2,30–35] The presence of multiple risk factors can increase the chances of AUS erosion even further to 25% to 75%.[31,35]

One of the worst complications that can occur after an AUS erosion is segmental urethral loss and resultant fibrosis or stricture formation (**Fig. 3**). The rates of urethral stricture may be influenced by AUS erosion management decisions. The options at the time of urethral erosion include urinary drainage alone (usually with placement of a urethral catheter) versus urethral repair in an effort to prevent urethral stricture or fistulization from the injured area. The group from UT Southwestern retrospectively described their experience with AUS erosion management.[36] Thirteen men were treated with catheter placement alone versus 13 men who underwent an in situ urethroplasty. The in situ urethroplasty involved suture repair of the ventral portion of the urethra, where erosions are usually most severe, and avoiding mobilization of the dorsal urethra. The investigators found a dramatic decrease in stricture formation, from 85% in the catheter-only group to 38% in the in situ urethroplasty group. Given that this was not a randomized study, there may be selection bias. In situ closure may not be possible for some erosions, such as shown in **Fig. 3**. In a similar study, investigators from the Cleveland Clinic studied the management of AUS erosion and subsequent stricture formation.[37] They grouped men into (1) treatment with catheter alone; (2) abbreviated urethroplasty, which is the same idea as the in situ urethroplasty; and (3) full anastomotic urethroplasty. The study was limited because most patients had catheter drainage (70%) compared with the 2 types of urethroplasty repair. The analysis (at 3 months' follow-up) included only 3 men who underwent abbreviated urethroplasty and 8 men who underwent anastomotic urethroplasty. In contrast with the study by UT Southwestern, this Cleveland Clinic study showed that stricture formation was higher in the urethroplasty groups. The stricture rate was 17% in the catheter drainage group, versus 33% in the abbreviated urethroplasty and 25% in the anastomotic urethroplasty groups. The study applied a grading system for urethral erosions as severe versus mild based on having more than 50% of the circumference of the urethra being disrupted. In an analysis examining only severe erosions there was a significant difference between groups: 38% in the catheter-only group, versus 0% in the abbreviated urethroplasty group and 25% in the anastomotic urethroplasty group. However, the analysis was underpowered because there were only 7 total strictures in severely eroded patients between the 3 groups. The most important finding of the study was that, for patients with mild erosions, only 1 patient out of 22 (5%) developed stricture when treated with a urethral catheter alone.[37] This finding suggests that stratifying the degree of damage is important to allow for identification of men who will reliably heal with a catheter alone versus those who need some type of urethral repair.

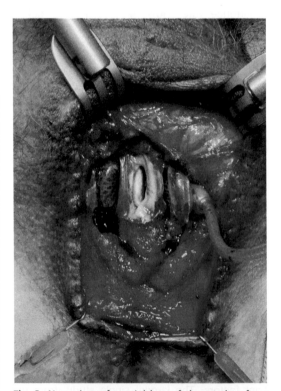

Fig. 3. Near circumferential loss of the urethra from severe erosion in a patient after radiotherapy, and anastomotic urethroplasty for rectourethral fistula, despite transcorporal AUS placement.

Future Questions About Urethral Stricture Management After Artificial Urinary Sphincter Erosion

To date, there have been no studies on the success of urethroplasty for urethral stricture when it does occur after AUS erosion and then the subsequent successful rate of AUS reimplantation.

Understanding the outcomes in this selected population of patients is important. If the outcomes are worse for AUS reimplantation compared with other well-known erosion risk factors, then surgeons would be more likely to recommend urethral closure and some type of urinary diversion, such as a suprapubic cystotomy, or other options. This possibility would avoid the unfortunate cycle of urethroplasty, reimplantation, and subsequent erosion and explantation. For instance, the patient shown in **Fig. 3** had successful closure of a rectourethral fistula, but was a smoker with emphysema and had a history of radiotherapy for prostate cancer. His urethra eroded within 3 months of placement of the AUS, which was placed in a transcorporal fashion. The urethra was successfully mobilized for anastomotic urethroplasty, but an intraoperative decision was made to close the urethra and rely on a suprapubic cystotomy because of his overall clinical condition. Data-driven decisions are important and can guide surgeons about how best to manage these types of difficult situations, which often arise in these patients.

ARTIFICIAL URINARY SPHINCTER PLACEMENT AFTER URETHRAL RECONSTRUCTION OR URETHROPLASTY

Some bladder neck contractures after radical prostatectomy and membranous strictures do not respond to endoscopic management. In these cases, reconstructive urologists have been developing successful strategies for open repair.[38,39] Bladder neck contractures can be approached from the abdomen, which can spare the membranous sphincter and preserve continence; however, this approach can require pubectomy because of the inferiorly recessed vesicourethral anastomosis and most men have already been rendered incontinent from previous endoscopic management. The same inferiorly recessed vesicourethral anastomosis lends itself to perineal repair, as does urethral strictures in the membranous urethra after radiotherapy. In this circumstance, the membranous urethral sphincter is almost certainly destroyed if it was not already in the fibrotic process of repetitive endoscopic management. In a perineal approach the bulbar urethra is mobilized, usually along most of its length. Urethral mobilization is necessary to bridge large gaps created by resection of scar and to remove irradiated urethra to create a healthy anastomosis to the prostate apex for membranous strictures after radiotherapy. Most often, the bulbar arteries are transected, or already destroyed from fibrosis, and the urethra relies solely on retrograde flow and perforators arising from the penile arteries.

Theoretically, the placement of an AUS obstructs retrograde blood flow through the urethra, and could cause the interval segment between the AUS and the more proximal anastomosis to become ischemic. Also, the urethra is usually atretic and is densely adhesed in the perineum from the previous surgery. In sum, these anatomic and surgical factors, after urethral reconstruction, make this subset of patients the most challenging for successful AUS implantation.

Outcomes of Artificial Urinary Sphincter Placement After Urethroplasty

There are few data on this complex patient group. Duke University published a small series of men who had successful rectourethral fistula repair, had incontinence, and had placement of an AUS.[40] Rectourethral fistula can be repaired by a variety of methods. For a simple fistula, closure of the fistula or the use of a buccal mucosa graft with a gracilis flap is very successful.[41] Alternatively, when there is concomitant membranous urethral stricture, as is often the case, anastomotic urethroplasty can also be used to resolve the fistula. In the series from Duke, rectourethral fistulas were all repaired without urethral mobilization. Thus the urethra may not be expected to be compromised as much as an anastomotic urethroplasty; even so, rectourethral fistula closure has a profound impact on urethral blood supply and postoperative fibrosis in the perineum. All the patients in this series had successful perineal placement of an AUS and did not require transcorporal placement or revision or explantation at 43 months' median follow-up.[40]

In another small series, investigators reported on 6 men undergoing anastomotic urethroplasty in which the urethral blood flow was expected to be compromised.[42] The causes of the strictures were split between BPE treatment and bladder neck contracture caused by radical prostatectomy. No patients had radiotherapy. Anastomotic urethroplasty was successful in all 6 patients and at 7 months after urethroplasty AUS placement was performed transperineally and without using a transcorporal approach. In these men, AUS placement was successful using a 4.0-cm cuff, and 1 man (17%) had an erosion within 6 months of implantation. No restenosis of the anastomotic repairs occurred.[42]

Two larger series studying erosion risk and AUS use in compromised urethras also addressed posturethroplasty AUS placement. TURNS published a study with an analysis of risk factors for AUS explantation (including infection, erosion, atrophy) and, at least in the short term (mean 2.3 years' follow-up), the explantation rate was only 4%. Specifically, there was 1 explanted case out of 28 men with a history of prior urethroplasty (3.6%).[31] Details of the urethroplasties were not available, but most of these were likely for membranous urethral stricture, or previous AUS erosion. UCSF recently published a similar study of a cohort of mostly high-risk men with compromised urethras, based on history of radiotherapy, previous AUS, and urethroplasty.[35] They reported on a total of 23 men who all underwent membranous anastomotic urethroplasty and found, at a median follow-up of 39 months, that the explantation rate for erosion, infection, or atrophy was 9 out of 23 (39%). Many of the 23 men had multiple compromising factors, such as radiation and a urethroplasty. A subanalysis of men with only 1 risk factor compared erosion risk between urethroplasty, radiation, and previous AUS and found that urethroplasty trended toward a worse risk factor compared with prior radiation treatment or AUS placement. Specifically, 44% of men with urethroplasty experienced erosion compared with 29% and 20% of men with radiation treatment or prior AUS, respectively.[35]

Transcorporal Artificial Urinary Sphincter Placement After Urethroplasty

After urethroplasty, many surgeons advocate transcorporal placement of AUS in order to diminish the risk of dorsal erosion, and increase the safety of placement of the AUS around a densely fibrotic postsurgical urethra. This technique was popularized by Webster at Duke University, but little has been written about its merits or risks.[43] Essentially a large flap of the tunica albuginea of the ventral corporal bodies is raised, starting lateral to the urethra. The flap makes it unnecessary to dissect the urethra off the corporal bodies and provides bulk to the dorsal urethra (**Fig. 4**).

A small retrospective series from UCSF compared men (n = 8) after transcorporal AUS placement with men undergoing standard AUS placement (n = 18).[44] Approximately 50% of men in both approaches had a history of radiotherapy, but 89% of men in the transcorporal arm of the study had 2 or more previous urethral procedures (including 5 out of 8 cases of anastomotic urethroplasty) compared with only 22% undergoing standard placement. At a follow-up of about 2 years, men undergoing standard placement had AUS explantation for erosion or infection twice as often (28%) as those undergoing transcorporal placement (13%). Despite the limitations caused by small numbers and disparate groups, the results support transcorporal placement. In another study on transcorporal placement from Vanderbilt, 35 men had transcorporal placement of AUS cuffs.[45] Unlike the previously mentioned UCSF study, there was no comparison group, but the investigators noted again that all of the erosions occurred in men with 2 or more urethral risk factors.[45] The TURNS network currently is conducting a trial with 12 centers randomizing men to transcorporal versus standard AUS placement.

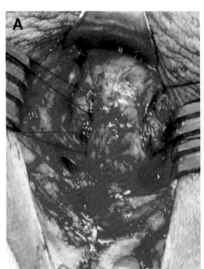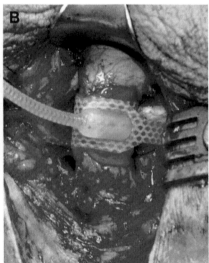

Fig. 4. Transcorporal AUS placement. Corporotomies are created on either side of the urethra with stay sutures that will be passed under the flap of tunica albuginea and tied as a horizontal mattress suture closing the corporal defect (*A*). The AUS placed around the urethra and the dorsal strip of tunica albuginea (*B*). (*Courtesy of* Sean Elliott, MD, Minneapolis, MN.)

Men being studied have a history of radiotherapy for prostate cancer and have not had AUS placement or other urethra-specific risk factors, such as a history of urethroplasty. It is hoped that this study will shed some light on the potential benefits of transcorporal placement (https://clinicaltrials.gov/ct2/show/NCT02524366).

SUMMARY

Urethral stricture and bladder neck contracture are among the most common issues that need to be addressed when AUS placement is being considered. Endoscopic management of bladder neck contracture has well-established outcomes and, depending on successful healing, an AUS can be placed safely afterward. If there is complete obliteration of the bladder neck or membranous stricture after radiotherapy, then abdominal bladder neck revision or perineal urethroplasty are very successful options. After urethroplasty, patients are at high risk for AUS erosion, but many can be managed successfully and, despite anatomic concerns about devascularization, there is little risk of proximal urethral necrosis in the limited series available to date. Erosions of the urethra resulting from an AUS can be a difficult complication; lower risk erosions that do not involve more than 50% of the circumference of the urethra can be managed with closure of the ventral defect or catheter drainage with modest risk of subsequent stricture. Alternatively, severe erosions probably benefit from an anastomotic urethroplasty when possible. There are no data on replacement of an AUS after urethroplasty for strictures arising from AUS urethral erosions. Transcorporal AUS placement, after urethroplasty or in compromised urethras, can avoid urethral injury and may decrease erosions rates, and many reconstructive surgeons (including the authors) believe this is an essential surgical step. An ongoing multicenter randomized clinical trial is accruing patients, and should give good data about transcorporal AUS placement in the subset of patients with a history of pelvic radiotherapy.

SUMMARY: KEY POINTS

- Bladder neck contracture can often be resolved with endoscopic treatment, and incontinence can be treated by AUS placement.
- Patients with complete obliteration of the bladder neck or with recalcitrant strictures can be treated successfully with open repair.
- Mild urethral erosions can be treated by catheter drainage or ventral urethral repair, whereas severe erosions should be repaired to prevent subsequent urethral stricture.
- AUS placement after urethroplasty is a risk factor for urethral erosion, but ischemic necrosis of the urethra is not common and in most cases AUS placement works well.

REFERENCES

1. Van der Aa F, Drake MJ, Kasyan GR, et al. The artificial urinary sphincter after a quarter of a century: a critical systematic review of its use in male non-neurogenic incontinence. Eur Urol 2013;63(4):681–9.
2. Wang R, McGuire EJ, He C, et al. Long-term outcomes after primary failures of artificial urinary sphincter implantation. Urology 2012;79(4):922–8.
3. Sandhu JS, Maschino AC, Vickers AJ. The surgical learning curve for artificial urinary sphincter procedures compared to typical surgeon experience. Eur Urol 2011;60(6):1285–90.
4. Jarosek SL, Virnig BA, Chu H, et al. Propensity-weighted long-term risk of urinary adverse events after prostate cancer surgery, radiation, or both. Eur Urol 2015;67(2):273–80.
5. Nam RK, Cheung P, Herschorn S, et al. Incidence of complications other than urinary incontinence or erectile dysfunction after radical prostatectomy or radiotherapy for prostate cancer: a population-based cohort study. Lancet Oncol 2014;15(2):223–31.
6. Elliott SP, Meng MV, Elkin EP, et al. Incidence of urethral stricture after primary treatment for prostate cancer: data From CaPSURE. J Urol 2007;178(2):529–34 [discussion: 534].
7. Carlsson S, Nilsson AE, Schumacher MC, et al. Surgery-related complications in 1253 robot-assisted and 485 open retropubic radical prostatectomies at the Karolinska University Hospital, Sweden. Urology 2010;75(5):1092–7.
8. Webb DR, Sethi K, Gee K. An analysis of the causes of bladder neck contracture after open and robot-assisted laparoscopic radical prostatectomy. BJU Int 2009;103(7):957–63.
9. Breyer BN, Davis CB, Cowan JE, et al. Incidence of bladder neck contracture after robot-assisted laparoscopic and open radical prostatectomy. BJU Int 2010;106(11):1734–8.
10. Jacobsen A, Berg KD, Iversen P, et al. Anastomotic complications after robot-assisted laparoscopic and open radical prostatectomy. Scand J Urol 2016;50(4):274–9.
11. Tang Y, Li J, Pu C, et al. Bipolar transurethral resection versus monopolar transurethral resection for benign prostatic hypertrophy: a systematic review and meta-analysis. J Endourol 2014;28(9):1107–14.

12. Montague DK, Angermeier KW, Paolone DR. Long-term continence and patient satisfaction after artificial sphincter implantation for urinary incontinence after prostatectomy. J Urol 2001;166(2):547–9.

13. Yurkanin JP, Dalkin BL, Cui H. Evaluation of cold knife urethrotomy for the treatment of anastomotic stricture after radical retropubic prostatectomy. J Urol 2001;165(5):1545–8.

14. Liberman D, Jarosek S, Virnig BA, et al. The patient burden of bladder outlet obstruction after prostate cancer treatment. J Urol 2016;195(5):1459–63.

15. Vanni AJ, Zinman LN, Buckley JC. Radial urethrotomy and intralesional mitomycin C for the management of recurrent bladder neck contractures. J Urol 2011;186(1):156–60.

16. Redshaw JD, Broghammer JA, Smith TG 3rd, et al. Intralesional injection of mitomycin C at transurethral incision of bladder neck contracture may offer limited benefit: TURNS study group. J Urol 2015; 193(2):587–92.

17. Brede C, Angermeier K, Wood H. Continence outcomes after treatment of recalcitrant postprostatectomy bladder neck contracture and review of the literature. Urology 2014;83(3):648–52.

18. Ramirez D, Zhao LC, Bagrodia A, et al. Deep lateral transurethral incisions for recurrent bladder neck contracture: promising 5-year experience using a standardized approach. Urology 2013;82(6):1430–5.

19. Biardeau X, Aharony S, AUS Consensus Group, et al. Artificial urinary sphincter: report of the 2015 consensus conference. Neurourol Urodyn 2016; 35(Suppl 2):S8–24.

20. Hussain M, Greenwell TJ, Shah J, et al. Long-term results of a self-expanding wallstent in the treatment of urethral stricture. BJU Int 2004;94(7):1037–9.

21. De Vocht TF, van Venrooij GE, Boon TA. Self-expanding stent insertion for urethral strictures: a 10-year follow-up. BJU Int 2003;91(7):627–30.

22. Buckley JC, Zinman LN. Removal of endoprosthesis with urethral preservation and simultaneous urethral reconstruction. J Urol 2012;188(3):856–60.

23. Eisenberg ML, Elliott SP, McAninch JW. Preservation of lower urinary tract function in posterior urethral stenosis: selection of appropriate patients for urethral stents. J Urol 2007;178(6):2456–60 [discussion: 2460–1].

24. Eisenberg ML, Elliott SP, McAninch JW. Management of restenosis after urethral stent placement. J Urol 2008;179(3):991–5.

25. Erickson BA, McAninch JW, Eisenberg ML, et al. Management for prostate cancer treatment related posterior urethral and bladder neck stenosis with stents. J Urol 2011;185(1):198–203.

26. Breyer BN, McAninch JW. Management of recalcitrant bladder neck contracture after radical prostatectomy for prostate cancer. Endoscopic and open surgery. J Urol 2011;185(2):390–1.

27. McNamara ER, Webster GD, Peterson AC. The Uro-Lume stent revisited: the Duke experience. Urology 2013;82(4):933–6.

28. Magera JS Jr, Inman BA, Elliott DS. Outcome analysis of urethral wall stent insertion with artificial urinary sphincter placement for severe recurrent bladder neck contracture following radical prostatectomy. J Urol 2009;181(3):1236–41.

29. Anger JT, Raj GV, Delvecchio FC, et al. Anastomotic contracture and incontinence after radical prostatectomy: a graded approach to management. J Urol 2005;173(4):1143–6.

30. Linder BJ, de Cogain M, Elliott DS. Long-term device outcomes of artificial urinary sphincter reimplantation following prior explantation for erosion or infection. J Urol 2014;191(3):734–8.

31. Brant WO, Erickson BA, Elliott SP, et al. Risk factors for erosion of artificial urinary sphincters: a multicenter prospective study. Urology 2014;84(4): 934–8.

32. Seideman CA, Zhao LC, Hudak SJ, et al. Is prolonged catheterization a risk factor for artificial urinary sphincter cuff erosion? Urology 2013;82(4): 943–6.

33. Ahyai SA, Ludwig TA, Dahlem R, et al. Outcomes of single versus double cuff artificial urinary sphincter insertion in low and high risk profile male patients with severe stress urinary incontinence. BJU Int 2016;114(4):625–32.

34. Raj GV, Peterson AC, Webster GD. Outcomes following erosions of the artificial urinary sphincter. J Urol 2006;175(6):2186–90 [discussion: 2190].

35. McGeady JB, McAninch JW, Truesdale MD, et al. Artificial urinary sphincter placement in compromised urethras and survival: a comparison of virgin, radiated and reoperative cases. J Urol 2014;192(6): 1756–61.

36. Rozanski AT, Tausch TJ, Ramirez D, et al. Immediate urethral repair during explantation prevents stricture formation after artificial urinary sphincter cuff erosion. J Urol 2014;192(2):442–6.

37. Chertack N, Chaparala H, Angermeier KW, et al. Foley or fix: a comparative analysis of reparative procedures at the time of explantation of artificial urinary sphincter for cuff erosion. Urology 2016;90:173–8.

38. Hofer MD, Zhao LC, Morey AF, et al. Outcomes after urethroplasty for radiotherapy induced bulbomembranous urethral stricture disease. J Urol 2014; 191(5):1307–12.

39. Glass AS, McAninch JW, Zaid UB, et al. Urethroplasty after radiation therapy for prostate cancer. Urology 2012;79(6):1402–5.

40. Selph JP, Madden-Fuentes R, Peterson AC, et al. Long-term artificial urinary sphincter outcomes following a prior rectourethral fistula repair. Urology 2015;86(3):608–12.

41. Vanni AJ, Buckley JC, Zinman LN. Management of surgical and radiation induced rectourethral fistulas with an interposition muscle flap and selective buccal mucosal onlay graft. J Urol 2010;184(6):2400–4.

42. Simonato A, Gregori A, Lissiani A, et al. Two-stage transperineal management of posterior urethral strictures or bladder neck contractures associated with urinary incontinence after prostate surgery and endoscopic treatment failures. Eur Urol 2007;52(5): 1499–504.

43. Guralnick ML, Miller E, Toh KL, et al. Transcorporal artificial urinary sphincter cuff placement in cases requiring revision for erosion and urethral atrophy. J Urol 2002;167(5):2075–8 [discussion: 2079].

44. Aaronson DS, Elliott SP, McAninch JW. Transcorporal artificial urinary sphincter placement for incontinence in high-risk patients after treatment of prostate cancer. Urology 2008; 72(4):825–7.

45. Mock S, Dmochowski RR, Brown ET, et al. The impact of urethral risk factors on transcorporeal artificial urinary sphincter erosion rates and device survival. J Urol 2015;194(6):1692–6.

Management of Urethral Strictures After Hypospadias Repair

Warren T. Snodgrass, MD, Nicol C. Bush, MD*

KEYWORDS

- Strictures after hypospadias repair • Hypospadias complications
- Reoperative hypospadias urethroplasty

KEY POINTS

- Strictures of the neourethra after hypospadias surgery are more common after skin flap repairs than urethral plate or neo-plate tubularizations.
- The diagnosis of stricture after hypospadias repair is suspected based on symptoms of stranguria, urinary retention, and/or urinary tract infection. It is confirmed by urethroscopy during anticipated repair, without preoperative urethrography.
- The most common repairs for neourethra stricture after hypospadias surgery are single-stage dorsal inlay graft and 2-stage labial mucosa replacement urethroplasty.
- The fact that a few adults present with strictures after childhood hypospadias repair does not imply that puberty or sexual activity causes deterioration of the neourethra, or that hypospadias is a lifelong problem.

PREVALENCE

Fifteen years ago, during the peak of preputial flap hypospadias repairs, urethral strictures were reported as a common complication, occurring in approximately 8% of cases. For example, Duel and colleagues[1] found 38 (7%) of 582 repairs resulted in a stricture following a variety of mostly skin flap or skin graft operations for predominantly proximal hypospadias. Weiner and colleagues[2] found strictures in 9% of patients after tubularized preputial flap repair, versus none using onlay preputial flaps. Two series of Byars' preputial flap repairs published this year reported urethral strictures in 8% and 12%.[3,4]

After Tubularizing the Urethral Plate

In contrast, procedures tubularizing the urethral plate (TIP) or a graft neoplate (2-stage preputial or oral mucosa graft repairs) have almost anecdotal prevalences of urethral strictures. For example, the authors reported no strictures in 426 consecutive distal hypospadias repairs with follow-up, all corrected using TIP.[5] They subsequently published urethral stricture occurring in 1 of 24 patients with proximal TIP who had mobilization of the urethral plate and proximal normal urethra for penile straightening.[6] Further analysis of those patients undergoing this dissection to correct penile curvature without transecting the urethral plate showed that nearly 20% developed focal, symptomatic strictures that did not occur in proximal TIP repairs without dissection under the urethral plate and urethra, and so that maneuver is no longer performed or recommended.

A meta-analysis of TIP complications that included primary distal and proximal, and reoperative, series reported the mean percentage of

PARC Urology, 5680 Frisco Square Boulevard, Suite 2300, Frisco, TX 75034, USA
* Corresponding author. 5680 Frisco Square Boulevard, Suite 2300, Frisco, TX 75034.
E-mail address: bush@parcurology.com

Urol Clin N Am 44 (2017) 105–111
http://dx.doi.org/10.1016/j.ucl.2016.08.014
0094-0143/17/© 2016 Elsevier Inc. All rights reserved.

reported urethral strictures was 1.3, 2.0, and 3.0, respectively.[7]

After 2-Stage Graft Repairs

Urethral strictures after primary 2-stage graft procedures, mostly using prepuce, did not occur in any patient in a series of 34 boys reported by Ferro and colleagues[8] or in the authors' series of 55 consecutive cases of severe hypospadias, defined as having ventral curvature greater than 30° after degloving.[9]

The authors also reported no urethral strictures in 45 patients undergoing 2-stage oral mucosa graft salvage repairs of hypospadias cripples, defined as patients undergoing reoperation for ventral curvature greater than 30°, grossly scarred urethral plate or skin, hairy neourethras, obliterative strictures or meatal stenosis, and/or balanitis xerotica obliterans.[10] Another similar series found urethral strictures in 16%, but did not further describe this observation,[11] which may have included meatal stenosis.

The low prevalence of strictures in TIP and 2-stage graft repairs suggests a higher incidence of technical error.

DIAGNOSIS

Strictures are most often diagnosed due to symptoms, including stranguria, urinary retention, and urinary tract infection, following hypospadias surgery. It is unusual to diagnose strictures in asymptomatic children, for example, on the basis of flow rate parameters alone.[1,6]

Uroflowmetry

Uroflowmetry was once recommended after hypospadias repair specifically to detect asymptomatic strictures. However, although Garibay and colleagues[12] emphasized a need for uroflowmetry after hypospadias repair, stating only 30% of patients diagnosed with obstruction had symptoms, only 2 of these patients had urethral strictures requiring repair. It is not clear from their article if these 2 had symptoms or not.

Meanwhile, studies of uroflows in patients with unoperated hypospadias report many have a Qmax around the fifth percentile of nomogram values and a plateau curve, likely indicating the formed urethra is also abnormal.[13] Therefore, postoperative urof_lometry with low Qmax and a plateau curve does not necessarily result from stricture, especially if the patient is otherwise asymptomatic.

Accordingly, many investigators have stated that uroflow parameters alone are not an indication

for invasive urethral studies.[14–17] The fact that Qmax tends to improve with time supports observation in asymptomatic patients with "obstructive" flow parameters after hypospadias repair.[16,17] This improvement in teens also argues against an increased risk for structuring during puberty.

Urethrography

Although an occasional patient with a stricture after hypospadias repair has a bulbar lesion, most often the obstruction is within the neourethra or at its junction to the native urethra. Although urethrography can be done, the relatively short distance from meatus to lesion in children, in contrast to adults, and the difficulty in holding the catheter in place while occluding the meatus in a moving child, who likely needs sedation, argues against this study. The authors never obtain this imaging.

Urethroscopy

Diagnosis of anatomic obstruction in children after hypospadias surgery is best done under general anesthesia, which facilitates accurate calibration of the neomeatus to rule out stenosis (<8 French), and urethroscopy to visualize a stricture.

MANAGEMENT
Dilations

There is no role for therapeutic dilations to manage urethral strictures in children.

Visual Urethrotomy

A protocol was followed to assess efficacy of visual urethrotomy (VU) to manage urethral strictures less than 1 cm in length after prior hypospadias surgery, with several important observations derived from a series of 72 patients.[18] Overall success, defined as symptom free at a minimum of 2 years of follow-up, with Qmax greater than 12 mL/s, was 24%.

Outcomes depended on the type of prior repair, with no success in 32 patients with tubularized grafts and 11% success in 18 with tubularized preputial flaps. In contrast, VU was successful in 72% of 11 with onlay preputial flaps and 63% of 11 with tubularized urethral plates.

Repeat VU was only done for recurrent strictures thought to still be less than 1 cm, with few successes (2/25) and nearly universal increase in subsequent length of the stricture. Rather than repeat VU, open urethroplasty was recommended for all recurrent strictures, even those still less than 1 cm.

Two other retrospective reviews of VU for post-hypospadias repair strictures also reported that repeat VU was not effective.[19,20] Therefore, if VU is selected for initial treatment of a posthypospadias repair stricture and is not successful, open urethroplasty should next be done.

Urethroplasty

Excision with anastomosis

The authors are not aware of published series regarding stricture excision with end-to-end anastomosis for lesions developing after hypospadias repair. They assume vascularity of neourethras is not as reliable as that of otherwise normal urethras affected by strictures and avoid this procedure, as do others.[21]

Instead, the authors choose between 1-stage dorsal oral mucosa graft inlay and 2-stage oral mucosa graft replacement urethroplasty for stricture repair.

One-stage graft inlay

Nonobliterative strictures usually can be corrected with a 1-stage inlay graft. Urethroscopy first confirms the stricture and its location. The meatus and neourethra distal to the stricture are calibrated to ensure normal caliber, which in children is greater than 8 French. Then, a ventral midline incision is made in the raphe. It is not necessary to deglove the penis.

The neourethra is opened ventrally proximal to the stricture and is then incised distally through the stricture and beyond a short distance, laying the stricture entirely open. If the stricture extends into the glans, then glans wings are developed and the neourethra is opened until healthy tissue is encountered or the meatus is open. Next, the dorsal midline of the neourethra and stricture is incised through the urethral wall, stopping just above the tunica albuginea of the corpora cavernosa. A 7-0 polydioxanone stay suture in the outer edge of the neourethra on each side holds the dorsal defect open until the graft is placed.

The defect is measured, and a graft of similar dimension is outlined on the inner surface of the upper lip, near the teeth. An inlay graft should not be taken from the lower lip, saving that site should recurrent stricture require a replacement urethroplasty. The mucosa is injected with bupivacaine mixed with 1:200,000 epinephrine, and then the borders of the graft are incised, beginning near the gums so that blood running down does not obscure the dissection. Next, the mucosa is dissected from the underlying fatty tissues and muscle, leaving behind as much fatty tissue as possible.

The authors leave gauze soaked in 1:1000 epinephrine against the harvest site. This gauze is removed at the end of the case, with additional hemostasis achieved using electrocautery as needed at that time. The donor site should not be sutured, but is left open for healing by secondary intention.

The graft is defatted. Larger grafts are best draped over the surgeon's finger to feel the pressure and depth of dissection. Smaller grafts will lay still for defatting by simply placing them onto a wet spot on the paper drape.

Then, the graft is sutured into the defect, beginning proximally and continuing with interrupted 7-0 polyglactin epithelial sutures around the perimeter distally. Both the proximal and the distal ends of the graft should enter well into normal neourethra beyond the stricture to reduce likelihood for recurrence.

The graft is finally quilted in the midline to secure it to the underlying corporal surface, using 7-0 polyglactin. The graft should be wide enough to stretch across the defect and affix to the corpora without tension; otherwise, the gain in width may not be sufficient.

A 6-French catheter is passed into the bladder. The ventral urethra is sutured using subepithelial stitches in 2 layers, as in a primary hypospadias urethroplasty. A flap of ventral dartos tissues is raised proximally and flipped up and over the entire repair to reduce risk for fistula. If there is not sufficient grossly healthy dartos, a tunica vaginalis flap can be harvested for a barrier layer.

Skin closure is done using interrupted subepithelial polyglactin. The catheter provides urinary diversion for approximately 10 days.

RESULTS

The largest published series of inlay grafts for hypospadias strictures was reported by Ye and colleagues,[22] involving 37 patients with a mean of 2 ± 1.8 (1-6) prior repairs. These patients were included in a series totaling 53. Mean inlay length was 4.6 ± 2.2 cm (3-7.5). Of the entire group, complications developed in 15% during a mean follow-up of 23 months. These complications comprised fistulas in 9% and recurrent strictures in 6%. All 3 recurrent strictures occurred at the proximal end.

Another report[23] included a total of 31 patients with a mean of 4 prior operations, of which half had strictures. The mean inlay length was 3.9 ± 2.5 cm (1-5), with the glans involved in 20 cases. Grafts were harvested from residual preduce, penile skin, or hairless groin skin rather than from the mouth. Complications occurred in

16% of patients, with proximal anastomotic strictures the most common.

As mentioned above, the primary repairs (TIP and 2-stage graft) that the authors use rarely result in stricture. Similarly, few patients referred to the authors with complications after repair elsewhere have isolated strictures. Of 367 hypospadias reoperations, only 15 (4%) had strictures as the major complication determining the surgical procedure (W. Snodgrass, N.C. Bush, 2016, unpublished data).

Of the authors' stricture operations, half had oral mucosa inlay graft repairs with no recurrent strictures. The authors suspect the proximal strictures reported by Ye and colleagues[22] and Schwentner and colleagues[23] may have resulted from not incising the dorsal neourethra sufficiently proximally to ensure that the end of the graft, which is relatively narrow and comes to a point, was in well-perfused tissues.

In the United States, most hypospadias operations include circumcision, and there is not sufficient skin at reoperation to harvest a graft or flap and still have sufficient skin to comfortably close the penile shaft without tension. Furthermore, these tissues were previously operated and so may have diminished vascularity. Accordingly, the authors prefer oral mucosa to add tissue for reoperative urethroplasty.

Two-Stage Oral Mucosa Graft

Indications for neourethral excision with 2-stage oral mucosa graft replacement urethroplasty include obliterative strictures (**Fig. 1**), and strictures associated with other complications including ventral curvature greater than 30°, hairy neourethra, and/or lichen sclerosus.

These reoperations can usually be approached through a ventral Y incision, re-creating glans wings and continuing down the median raphe. The neourethra is entirely excised distally to proximally until healthy native urethra is encountered. Scarred dartos and any remaining corpus spongiosum are also excised, leaving the surface of the corpora cavernosa exposed and clean.

A proximal urethrostomy is made by spatulating the native urethra ventrally and then suturing adjacent shaft or scrotal skin to 5, 6, and 7 o'clock using interrupted polyglactin.

Then, a throat pack is inserted to prevent blood from entering the esophagus, and the lower lip is exposed with stay sutures. A large graft is outlined approximately 2 mm inside the vermillion border of the lip, close to the gum, and into the junction with the cheek on each side (**Fig. 2**). It is then injected with bupivacaine with 1:200,000 epinephrine and harvested as discussed earlier.

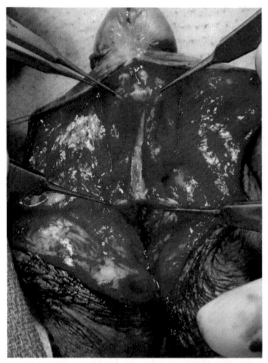

Fig. 1. Obliterative stricture of the hypospadias neourethra. The proximal aspect of the neourethra extending to at least the corona of the glans demonstrates a stricture that leaves an inadequate width of tissue for incision and inlay grafting. Therefore, excision of the entire neourethra with 2-stage labial mucosa replacement urethroplasty is needed. Patients with this extent of stricture after hypospadias repair may also have recurrent ventral curvature, which also requires excision of the neourethra to straighten.

The donor site is covered with gauze soaked in 1:1000 epinephrine while work continues on the penis. The wound in not sutured, because this will distort the external appearance.

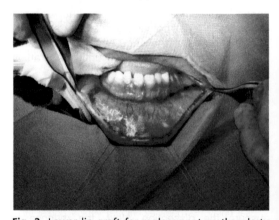

Fig. 2. Lower lip graft for replacement urethroplasty. This graft will provide sufficient tissue to extend in a single piece from the meatus to a scrotal urethrostomy in both children and adults. The donor site is not sutured.

After defatting, the graft is sutured into the widely opened glans wings and then proximally to shaft skin toward the urethrostomy using interrupted polyglactin. Distal stitches at the end of the glans are placed under the epithelium to avoid suture marks at the future neomeatus.

The graft is split proximally to extend to either side of the urethrostomy and then sutured at the 2, 12, and 10 o'clock positions to complete the stoma. Finally, the graft is quilted to the corpora at 0.5- to 1-cm intervals, first down the midline and then to either side, to reduce risk for hematoma or seroma accumulating underneath it.

A tie-over Vaseline gauze bandage provides gentle compression to the graft. This bandage and a catheter in the urethrostomy are removed 1 week later.

Second-stage tubularization is done 6 months later. Briefly, incision is made along the edge of the neourethral plate (the revascularized graft), re-creating glans wings, then extending into the urethrostomy to remove penile or scrotal skin from 5 to 7 o'clock, and finally, continuing in the scrotal midline for later access to tunica vaginalis.

The neo-plate is tubularized over a 6-French stent in prepubertal boys, or 12- to 14-French catheter in teens and adults. A 2-layer subepithelial closure is done beginning at approximately the midglans distally (to avoid meatal stenosis), the first layer using interrupted polyglactin, and the second layer using continuous polydioxanone.

Tunica vaginalis, rather than dartos, is used to cover the neourethra. Then glansplasty is done also beginning at approximately the midglans, placing 3 subepithelial polyglactin interrupted sutures between the glanular neomeatus and the corona. The glans wings are not sutured to the underlying tubularized neourethra.

Skin is approximated in the midline raphe with interrupted subepithelial sutures. Urinary diversion is maintained for 2 weeks.

Results: first stage

The authors reported 10% of patients undergoing 2-stage oral mucosa graft urethroplasty for salvage hypospadias repair (mean 4, range 1–20 prior operations) developed focal (n = 4) or complete (n = 1) graft contracture requiring an additional partial or complete graft procedure before the second stage.[10] The authors initially used cheek grafts and closed the donor site. These grafts created a thick neourethral plate that made glansplasty difficult, and so next, the authors made composite grafts, placing lip into the glans and cheek on the shaft.

Eventually, the authors learned that nearly any urethral defect can be replaced using only lower lip, and that harvesting the largest possible graft reduced the need to additional graft procedures. In the next 88 patients, graft reoperations were needed in only 4.[24] However, a recent review of adult stricture surgery included photographs of a 2-stage oral mucosa graft repair in which the glans was not opened widely and the graft was not made sufficiently wide to allow for postoperative shrinkage.[21]

Others have reported higher first-stage complication rates to 22%,[25] although of these, a similar 7% had graft contracture and 3% had urethrostomy stenosis.

Longitudinal graft contracture that results in ventral curvature greater than or equal to 30° requires partial or complete regrafting. Transverse partial contracture can often be overcome by either making the skin incision wider and incorporating healthy adjacent shaft skin with the oral mucosa into the neourethra or making a midline TIP-like incision for a dorsal inlay of additional oral mucosa.

The most important lessons the authors have learned are to use lower lip and to take the largest possible grafts.

Second stage

In the authors' series, 17 of 45 (38%) patients with follow-up had urethroplasty complications, mostly glans dehiscence and fistulas, which are common complications after hypospadias repair.[10] There were only 2 cases with meatal stenosis, and no strictures or diverticula. Similarly, Leslie and colleagues[11] reported 37% complications, with fistulas, glans dehiscence, and meatal stenosis, but no postoperative strictures.

Hypospadias Strictures Versus Strictures of Other Causes

Most hypospadias strictures occur in the anterior urethra, in the neourethra, or at its junction to the native urethra, in contrast to strictures from other causes, which are more common in the bulb. Occasionally, a patient with a hypospadias stricture in the neourethra will also be found to have a bulbar stricture, possibly from trauma related to instrumentation, but this is unusual. Preoperative imaging to rule out a more proximal stricture is not needed, because it will be found intraoperatively when an attempt is made to pass a catheter, and it can be managed simultaneously with a more distal obstruction.

The distal urethra in men with bulbar strictures most often is normal, and for that reason, can be mobilized to facilitate a primary anastomosis when the stricture is short. However, the neourethra after hypospadias repair is not a normal urethra, and the presence of a stricture implies a region of impaired vascularity. It is not advised to mobilize the neourethra as part of stricture excision and primary anastomosis, but rather repair by inlay graft or 2-stage grafting should be done as described earlier.

One reason for hypospadias repair is to facilitate voiding with a straight, compact stream. Teens and adults with uncorrected hypospadias in which the glans does not encircle the meatus often experience a deviated and/or spraying stream, which may cause them to sit to void. That, in turn, can be embarrassing and shameful. The authors' data indicate that hypospadias surgery, including reoperations, has the same outcome in both children and adults, meaning adults can be repaired with the same goals as children, including a meatus normally positioned in the glans.[26] There have been recommendations that men with distal obstruction from meatal stenosis or a neourethral stricture simply have the meatus cut open back to healthy urethra, but the authors believe this should be a rare consideration based mostly on comorbidities—rather than concern for healing in adults.

Strictures in Adults After Childhood Hypospadias Repair

Several recent publications[25,27,28] by adult reconstructive urologists call attention to complications in men after childhood hypospadias repair. Because adult specialists are known for stricture management, it is not surprising these patients referred to them mostly have strictures.

Most of these series are retrospective and accumulated patients over periods ranging from 6 to 30 years. The largest series included only 60 subjects. None report the technique used for primary repair in childhood, but most were done in the era of skin flaps before urethral plate tubularizations and staged graft repairs gained popularity.

The presentation of adults having strictures of the neourethra after childhood repair has led to speculation that these repairs may not be durable through puberty and the onset of sexual activity, especially when there is absence of the corpus spongiosum.[27] This idea implies that problems in adults are new problems and not lingering complications from their childhood surgery. That may be true of some strictures, although it can be difficult to determine their time of onset, whether they result from hypospadias surgery or are idiopathic.

The fact that a few men are diagnosed with strictures after childhood repair should not be generalized to recommendations regarding pediatric hypospadias surgery. First, each year in the United States, some 10,000 primary hypospadias repairs are done, yet recent articles concerning adults together comprise less than 150 subjects.[25,27,28] If there was a significant risk for deterioration of successful childhood repairs during pubertal development and sexual activity, one would expect thousands of men to present to adult specialists for management. In addition, as stated above, most the reported subjects likely had skin flap urethroplasties, which are done much less frequently today. Available uroflowmetry data from teens with childhood TIP repair show Qmax increasing during puberty,[16,17] which argues against stricturing.

Furthermore, the authors' practice involves hypospadias surgery in patients of all ages, and they systematically ask when symptoms first occurred. Rarely, a teen will report new onset of a fistula, but all the authors' patients with dehiscence, stenosis/stricture, and/or curvature stated these complications (or symptoms that led to their diagnosis) were present before puberty. In other words, the hypospadias complications the authors encounter in adults represent complications never corrected after childhood surgery.

Finally, if absence of corpus spongiosum predicts future stricture development, then modern repair by TIP should decrease that occurrence, because the spongiosum is preserved and sutured over the neourethra when the wings diverge. However, repair when curvature exceeds 30° after degloving requires urethral plate transection and a tubularized flap or 2-stage graft repair, which will not have spongiosum whether the surgery is done in children or adults. Childhood repair would still be recommended, because not all patients would eventually develop strictures, and surgery can be done by the surgeons most familiar with hypospadias repair at an age when most patients will not recall the operation.

What is most apparent is that men with primary hypospadias or complications after childhood repair are classified into a no-man's land between pediatric and adult specialists. The overwhelming majority of hypospadias surgery is performed by pediatric urologists, whose practices are usually limited to children. Adult specialists are experts in stricture repair, but are less familiar and practiced with hypospadias techniques. To bridge this gap, some specialists are needed who perform hypospadias surgery in both children and adults, meaning there is a need for greater cross-training and scientific exchange between pediatric and adult reconstructive urologists.

REFERENCES

1. Duel BP, Barthold JS, Gonzalez R. Management of urethral strictures after hypospadias repair. J Urol 1998;160:170–1.

2. Weiner JS, Sutherland RW, Roth DR, et al. Comparison of onlay and tubularized island flaps of inner preputial skin for the repair of proximal hypospadias. J Urol 1997;158:1172–4.

3. Stanasel I, Le HK, Bilgutay A, et al. Complications following staged hypospadias repair using transposed prepucial skin flaps. J Urol 2015; 194:512–6.

4. McNamara ER, Schaeffer AJ, Seager CM, et al. Management of proximal hypospadias with 2-stage repair: 20-year experience. J Urol 2015;194:1080–5.

5. Snodgrass WT, Bush N, Cost N. Tubularized incised plate hypospadias repair for distal hypospadias. J Pediatr Urol 2010;6:408–13.

6. Snodgrass WT, Granberg C, Bush NC. Urethral strictures following urethral plate and proximal urethral elevation during proximal TIP hypospadias repair. J Pediatr Urol 2013;9:990–4.

7. Pfistermuller KL, McArdle AJ, Cuckow PM. Meta-analysis of complication rates of the tubularized incised plate (TIP) repair. J Pediatr Urol 2015; 11:54–9.

8. Ferro F, Zaccara A, Spagnoli A, et al. Skin graft for 2-stage treatment of severe hypospadias: back to the future? J Urol 2002;168:1730–3.

9. Snodgrass W, Bush NC. 2-stage graft for primary proximal hypospadias with >30° ventral curvature. Abstract presented to ESPU, 2015.

10. Snodgrass WT, Bush N, Cost N. Algorithm for comprehensive approach to hypospadias reoperation using 3 techniques. J Urol 2009;182:2885–91.

11. Leslie B, Lorenzo AJ, Figueroa V, et al. Critical outcome analysis of staged buccal mucosa graft urethroplasty for prior failed hypospadias repair in children. J Urol 2011;185:1077–82.

12. Garibay JT, Reid C, Gonzalez R. Functional evaluation of the results of hypospadias surgery with uroflowmetry. J Urol 1995;154:835–6.

13. Maylon AD, Boorman JG, Blwley N. Urinary flow rates in hypospadias. Br J Plast Surg 1997;50:530–5.

14. Jayanthi VR, McLorie GA, Khoury AE, et al. Functional characteristics of the reconstructed neourethra after island flap urethroplasty. J Urol 1995; 153:1657–9.

15. Hammouda HM, El-Ghoneimi A, Bagli DJ, et al. Tubularized incised plate repair: functional outcome after intermediate followup. J Urol 2003;169:331–3.

16. Andersson M, Doroszkiewicz M, Arfwidsson C, et al. Hypospadias repair with tubularized incised plate: does the obstructive flow pattern resolve spontaneously? J Pediatr Urol 2010;7:441–5.

17. Hueber P, Antczac C, Abdo A, et al. Long-term functional outcomes of distal hypospadias repair: a single center retrospective comparative study of TIPs, Mathieu and MAGPI. J Pediatr Urol 2015;11:68.e1-7.

18. Husmann DA, Rathbun SR. Long-term follow up of visual internal urethrotomy for management of short (less than 1cm) penile urethral structures following hypospadias repair. J Urol 2006;176:1738–41.

19. Hsiao KC, Baez-Trinidad L, Lendvay T, et al. Direct vision internal urethrotomy for the treatment of pediatric urethral strictures: analysis of 50 patients. J Urol 2003;170:952–5.

20. Gargollo PC, Cai AW, Borer JG, et al. Management of recurrent urethral strictures after hypospadias repair: is there a role for repeat dilation or endoscopic incision? J Pediatr Urol 2011;7:34–8.

21. Craig JR, Wallis C, Brant WO, et al. Management of adults with prior failed hypospadias surgery. Transl Androl Urol 2014;3:196–204.

22. Ye WJ, Ping P, Liu YD, et al. Single stage dorsal inlay buccal mucosa graft with tubularized incised urethral plate technique for hypospadias reoperations. Asian J Androl 2008;10:682–6.

23. Schwentner C, Gozzi C, Lunacek A, et al. Interim outcome of the single stage dorsal inlay skin graft for complex hypospadias reoperations. J Urol 2006;175:1872–6.

24. Snodgrass W, Bush NC. Reoperative hypospadias urethroplasty. In: Hypospadiology. Frisco (TX): Operation Happenis; 2015. p. 155–70.

25. Kozinn SI, Harty NJ, Zinman L, et al. Management of complex anterior urethral strictures with multistage buccal mucosa graft reconstruction. Urology 2013; 82:718–22.

26. Snodgrass W, Villanueva C, Bush N. Primary and reoperative hypospadias repair in adults—are results different than in children? J Urol 2014;192:1730–3.

27. Barbagli G, de Angelis M, Palminteri E, et al. Failed hypospadias repair presenting in adults. Eur Urol 2006;49:887–94.

28. Myers JB, McAninch JW, Erickson BA, et al. Treatment of adults with complications from previous hypospadias surgery. J Urol 2012;188:459–63.

Urologic Sequelae Following Phalloplasty in Transgendered Patients

Dmitriy Nikolavsky, MD[a],*, Yuka Yamaguchi, MD[b],
Jamie P. Levine, MD[c], Lee C. Zhao, MD, MS[d]

KEYWORDS

- Urethral stricture • Fistula • Phalloplasty • Metoidioplasty • Transgender reconstruction
- Complications

KEY POINTS

- Urinary fistula and urethral stricture are common after neophallus reconstruction.
- Fistulas commonly occur at sites of anastomosis.
- Reconstruction must be tailored to the patient's anatomy and goals.

INTRODUCTION

In recent years, the issues of the transgender population have become more visible in the media worldwide. It has been estimated that approximately 355 individuals per 100,000 population consider themselves transgender or experience gender dysphoria to a varied degree, and approximately 9.8 per 100,000 would seek affirmation therapy.[1] Complete transformation to the new gender involves several pharmaceutical and surgical steps. Transgender patients at various stages of their transformation will present to urologic clinics requiring general or specialized urologic care. Knowledge of specifics of reconstructed anatomy and potential unique complications of the reconstruction will become important in providing urologic care to these patients.

Our review of literature combined with the authors' personal experience suggest that in patients undergoing male-to-female transformation, the genitourinary complications are uncommon: recto-neovaginal fistula (1%) and meatal stenosis (5%).[2,3] Thus, in this review, we have concentrated on describing the more common urologic complications after female-to-male reconstructions.

UROLOGIC ISSUES IN FEMALE-TO-MALE TRANSGENDER PATIENTS

One goal of neophallus construction in female-to-male transgender surgery is to achieve the ability for the individual to void while standing. Although some patients use external "urinary assist" devices from the native urethra to facilitate urination while standing,[4–6] many undergo neourethra construction, as the ability to stand to void is a high priority among female-to-male transgender individuals. More than 98% reported a desire to stand to void.[7] The management of urologic sequelae is important after neourethra construction, as

Disclosures: The authors have no financial or commercial conflicts of interests and no funding sources for this article.
[a] Department of Urology, Upstate University Hospital, SUNY Upstate Medical University, 750 East Adams Street, Syracuse, NY 13210, USA; [b] Division of Urology, Department of Surgery, Highland Hospital, Alameda Health System, 1411 East 31st Street, Oakland, CA 94602, USA; [c] Hansjörg Wyss Department of Plastic Surgery, New York University School of Medicine, 305 East 33rd Street, New York, NY 10016, USA; [d] Department of Urology, New York University School of Medicine, 150 East 32nd Street, 2nd Floor, New York, NY 10016, USA
* Corresponding author.
E-mail address: Nikolavd@upstate.edu

0094-0143/17/© 2016 Elsevier Inc. All rights reserved.

urologic.theclinics.com

fistulae, strictures, and persistent vaginal cavities are common complications.

ANATOMY OF METOIDIOPLASTY AND PHALLOPLASTY

Female-to-male transgender patients are typically offered 2 options for genital reconstruction: metoidioplasty versus phalloplasty. Metoidioplasty in its many forms involves lengthening of native urethra by means of local vaginal and labial flaps to create a neophallus long enough for urination in a standing position. The techniques are similar to proximal hypospadias repair in pediatric patients.[8] At the end of the operation, the labia minora is tubularized to form the distal urethra, the clitoris is freed from the attachments and elongated to form the glans, and the labia majora is used to create a neoscrotum and to cover the shaft of the neophallus. As a result, the urethra after metoidioplasty consists of 2 parts: the proximal native urethra with its meatus connected to a distal neourethra created from the labia minora.

Metoidioplasty is an attractive option for patients who would want to avoid more invasive phalloplasty options that involve distant tissue flaps and grafts. The complications are typically minor and may involve ventral fistulae, infrequent stricture at the level of neourethra, and remnant vaginal cavity. The main disadvantage of this procedure is limited length and girth of the resultant neophallus, precluding its use for intercourse.

In contrast, phalloplasty is offered to patients who desire to achieve both voiding and sexual functions. As expected, this is a more invasive option, involving a combination of local and distant tissue transfer techniques. The urethra of the male-to-female transgendered patient after phalloplasty can be divided into distinct segments,[6,9] from proximal to distal: native (female) urethra, fixed urethra, anastomotic urethra, phallic urethra, and meatus. The fixed urethra is the portion of the urethra formed after lengthening the native urethra via local vaginal or labial flaps, extragenital flaps, and grafts of skin or mucosa.[6,10] The phallic urethra can be constructed through a variety of techniques, including prelamination, prefabrication, tube-in-tube techniques, and pedicle flaps.[6,10]

FISTULA

Urethrocutaneous fistula is the most common urethral complication. The fistula rate of radial forearm free flap phalloplasty ranges from 22% to 75%.[11–14] Urethral fistulas commonly occur at points of anastomosis: between the phallic urethra and fixed urethra, and between the fixed urethra

and the native urethra, although fistulae can occur anywhere along the neourethra.[15] Fistulas occur most commonly at or just proximal to the anastomosis between the phallic urethra and fixed urethra[12] due to vascular insufficiency of the flap, and the decreased lumen of the phallic urethra. The change in caliber of the lumen from fixed to phallic urethra may cause a relative obstruction of the urinary stream distal to the site of the fistula.[12] The small-caliber lumen of the phallic urethra may be due to tissue shrinkage or insufficient size of the urethra at the time of construction. Spontaneous closure of the fistula tract has been reported, with Fang and colleagues[16] reporting spontaneous closure of the fistula within 2 months in as many as 35.7% of patients.

PERSISTENT VAGINAL CAVITY

In our combined experience, fistulae proximal to the anastomosis commonly communicate with large remnant vaginal cavities and are unlikely to close spontaneously if there is distal obstruction (**Fig. 1**). We suspect that in the presence of distal obstruction, pressurized urine finds its way through the ventral suture lines of the fixed urethra and into the obliterated vaginal cavity after previous vaginectomy or colpocleisis. If this persistent cavity is found, we routinely perform complete cavity excision and obliteration at the time of the fistula repair. Surprisingly, in our experience, pathologic analysis showed normal vaginal epithelium in all cavity specimens, despite the previous history of vaginectomy.

STRICTURE

Urethral stricture is another common urologic complication with reports of incidence varying from 25% to 58%.[12,17,18] Although stricture can occur in any segment of the urethra, the most common location of stricture formation is at the anastomosis of the fixed and phallic portion of the neourethra (**Fig. 2**). Lumen and colleagues[9] characterized stricture formation after phalloplasty and determined that urethral stricture occurred at the anastomosis in 40.7%, phallic portion in 28%, the meatus in 15.3%, fixed segment in 12.7%, and multifocal in 7.6%. Ischemia is thought to be the etiology of strictures at all levels. Fistula formation also may contribute to dense scar formation and kinking of the tissues, especially at the anastomosis of the phallic to fixed portions.[9,17] At the meatus, contracture of the anastomosis between the skin of the glans and the neourethral tissue can lead to meatal stenosis. Mean stricture length in this series was 3.6 cm (range: 0.5–15 cm).[9] Fistula and urethral

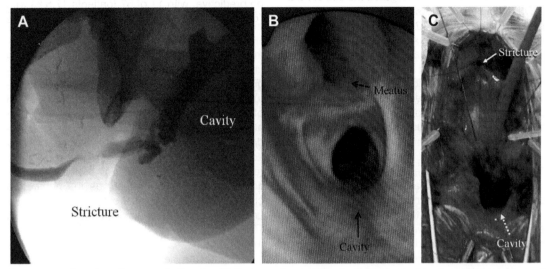

Fig. 1. Examples of persistent vaginal cavity. (*A*) Retrograde urethrogram of patient with anastomotic stricture of the neophallic urethra and large persistent vaginal cavity. (*B*) Cystoscopic view of remnant vaginal cavity (*below*) and native urethral meatus (*above*). (*C*) Intraoperative view of another patient with both anastomotic stricture and persistent vaginal cavity (urethral catheter is seen in native urethral meatus).

stricture may occur simultaneously. In a series of 1-stage urethroplasty by Rohrmann and Jaske,[12] 40% of patients developed fistula and strictures, with the fistula usually proximal to the stricture.

Proper management of urologic sequelae of phalloplasty is mandatory given that urinary fistulae and urinary obstruction due to urethral stricture can have grave consequences, such as chronic infection, sepsis, and renal failure, as well as compromised quality of life. If the patient is in urinary retention, urinary drainage must be performed, with placement of a suprapubic catheter. The extent of subsequent urinary reconstruction will depend on the individual's health and preferences.

PATIENT EVALUATION

A patient with urologic sequelae after phalloplasty will often present with voiding complaints. This may include increased difficulty with urination, whether with decreased stream or increased need to strain to void, or a complete inability to void. If a urethrocutaneous fistula has formed, the patient may complain of urine or purulent drainage at a location other than the meatus. The drainage may occur at the time of micturition but may also occur afterward due to pooling of the urine in the urinary tract or persistent vaginal cavity. The patient may also complain of dysuria or suprapubic pain.

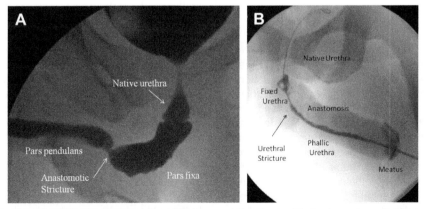

Fig. 2. (*A*) Combined voiding and retrograde urethrograms of patient with short anastomotic stricture of a neophallic urethra. The location of the stricture is at the junction of fixed urethra and phallic urethra. (*B*) Retrograde urethrogram of patient with neophallus showing extensive penile stricture from anastomosis to neomeatus.

The first step in patient evaluation is careful physical examination. The suprapubic area and neophallus should be examined for evidence of infection, such as erythema and induration. The areas are also palpated for fluctuance to determine if there are any fluid collections that require drainage. Ultrasound may be performed to evaluate for the presence of an abscess. All areas are evaluated for fistulous openings, and the urethral meatus itself is examined for patency.

Infections should be treated before surgery. Cellulitis should be treated. If there is concern for urinary tract infection, a urine sample may be sent for urinalysis and urine culture. If the patient has a suprapubic tube, the urine sample may be sent from the tube. Indwelling catheters are often colonized, however, and organisms grown from these cultures may not be representative of infections. If the urine culture returns positive with clinical indication of infection, then culture-specific antibiotics should be given.

Suprapubic tenderness and flank pain can be the result of urinary retention and an overly distended bladder. A postvoid residual can be determined using a bladder scanner. If the patient is in urinary retention, drainage of the bladder should be performed. As the patient typically has a urethral stricture that precludes urethral catheterization, a suprapubic tube should be placed to ensure adequate urinary drainage.

Further anatomic evaluation can be performed via both retrograde urethrogram and if possible, voiding cystourethrogram to help delineate the location of the stricture or fistula. Examination under anesthesia is frequently useful given the complex urinary anatomy of a patient status post phalloplasty. A suprapubic tube can be placed at the time of this examination if the patient does not already have one in place.

PREOPERATIVE PLANNING AND PREPARATION

Notation should be taken as to the patient's previous surgeries and what potential flaps and grafts are available for use for urologic reconstruction.

The first step in managing a urinary fistula or stricture causing urinary obstruction would be to ensure that the patient's urine is adequately diverted with a suprapubic catheter of adequate size. The suprapubic catheter should be placed 2 to 4 cm above the pubis. Placement of a 16-French or larger catheter facilitates the use of the suprapubic channel for antegrade cystourethroscopy to delineate the proximal urethra. Antegrade cystourethroscopy is easiest when the suprapubic tube is at the midline. Care must be

taken to avoid damage to the vascular anastomosis to the neophallus.

The standard preoperative evaluation for urethral strictures and fistulae includes a retrograde urethrogram combined with antegrade and retrograde endoscopy to determine the extent of stricture and evaluate for presence of fistulization and pelvic cavity. The patient is brought to the operating room and the patient is placed in low lithotomy position and prepped and draped to allow access to the perineum as well as the suprapubic region. A layer of complexity is added in the patient status post phalloplasty as the neourethra created may be of a smaller caliber than the native urethra and unable to accommodate a standard 16-French flexible cystourethroscope. At the authors' institutions, we use a flexible ureteroscope to navigate the neourethra. The retrograde urethrogram can be performed by injecting contrast via the ureteroscope. This technique has the advantage of allowing for direct visualization of the neourethra rather than attempting to blindly pass a catheter into a possibly tortuous neourethra. A guidewire is used to gradually advance the ureteroscope. Once contrast is injected, fluoroscopic images are obtained to delineate the anatomy of the stricture and fistulae. If the suprapubic tract is mature, antegrade cystoscopy may be performed to delineate the anatomy proximal to the stricture point. Location, length, and caliber of the stricture as well as location of any fistulae are key factors to determine. Any fluid collections or abscesses that have formed due to obstruction should be adequately drained. If a fistula does not heal on its own, often excision of the fistula tract with closure and coverage with a flap is required.

Before any reconstructive effort, the risks of each possible intervention should be discussed in detail with the patients, including risks from harvesting new flaps and grafts, and from performing urethroplasty, redo vaginectomy, or fistula repair. The possibility of multistage procedures should be discussed, as well as remote possibility of total or partial loss of the neophallus. The most important consideration in choice of reconstruction is the patient's preference and desire to void upright. Some may choose to avoid heroic reconstructive measures and may elect for the simpler option of perineal urethrostomy.

SURGICAL TECHNIQUES

The patient is placed under general anesthesia. Care is taken to position the endotracheal tube to the side opposite the potential side of graft harvest if a buccal graft is planned. Positioning the patient in lithotomy position allows access to the genitalia and suprapubic area, as well as the thighs as needed for flap harvest.

Fistulae

All procedures are performed with the assistance of antegrade and retrograde cystourethroscopy for delineation of anatomy. Due to the absence of normal landmarks within the neourethra, identification of the fistula site often requires simultaneous cystourethroscopy with exposure of the cutaneous fistula tract. A needle, guidewire, or a lacrimal duct probe inserted from the opening of the fistula into the urethral lumen is then visualized with the cystoscope and can be further used to identify the approximate distance and trajectory of the urethra from the skin surface. A "cut to the light" procedure can be performed, in which the fistula tract is dissected toward the light of the cystoscope. Concentric stay sutures placed at the edges of the tract may facilitate the excision. The fistula tract is excised and the opening to the urethra closed in multiple nonoverlapping layers. Consideration must be made for flap coverage of the site, to decrease the risk of fistula recurrence. We generally use a fasciocutaneous groin flap to cover the anastomosis (**Fig. 3**) or "recycle" a labial fat pad flap harvested from the neoscrotum. If a distal stricture is associated with the fistula, then the stricture must be repaired. Otherwise, high-pressure voiding due to obstruction will result in fistula recurrence. Likewise, if the communicating remnant pelvic cavity is present, it is to be meticulously excised and obliterated at the time of fistula repair.

Strictures

Management of urethral strictures in the female-to-male patient can be challenging. Endoscopic management with dilation and direct visualization internal urethrotomy (DVIU) have been prone to failure, with Levine and Elterman[17] reporting a restricture rate of 87.5% in patients who underwent endoscopic urethrotomy. The relative decrease in success rates of endoscopic management in neophalluses when compared with native urethras is likely secondary to lack of corpus spongiosum and otherwise poor blood supply. Lumen and colleagues,[19] however, reported that visual internal urethrotomy would be a reasonable first-line approach for shorter strictures less than 3 cm in length. First-time DVIU was successful in 43.8% with an additional 12.5% patent with a second DVIU at a median follow-up of 51 months (range: 8–95). Three or more endoscopic interventions were not successful. Of note, in their series, a Foley catheter was left in place for 2 weeks after the DVIU to allow for healing of the epithelium lining the urethra. Shorter time to stricture formation was a significant risk factor for failure of endoscopic intervention.[19]

In patients with longer or multifocal strictures, or in whom endoscopic management fails, urethroplasty must be performed. Approach to urethroplasty depends on location of the stricture and length of the affected segment (**Fig. 4**). Different types of urethroplasty used for the treatment of urethral strictures after phallic reconstructions include meatotomy, Heineke-Mikulicz principle, excision and primary anastomosis, free graft urethroplasty, pedicled flap urethroplasty, 2-stage urethroplasty, and perineal urethrostomy, which may be followed by urethral reconstruction.[9] If a penile prosthesis is present, the urethra is opened ventrally.[9]

Single-Stage Anastomotic Techniques

Shorter segments of stricture may not require additional graft or flap material. Meatal stenosis may be treated with meatotomy if the stenotic segment is short. This may result in a hypospadiac meatus. At our institutions, we prefer to cut the meatus both ventrally and dorsally to reduce the appearance of hypospadias. The hindered mobility of the urethral and glans tissue limits

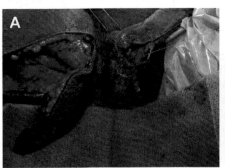
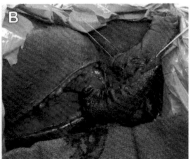

Fig. 3. Steps of single-stage urethroplasty with use of fasciocutaneous flap from the thigh. Urethroplasty performed by harvesting a fasciocutaneous flap (*A*) that is rotated up to cover the ventral aspect of the urethra (*B*).

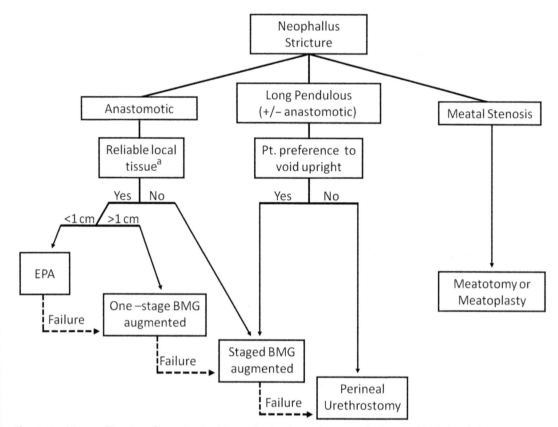

Fig. 4. Decision-making tree for patient with urethral stricture in a neophallus. [a]Reliable local tissue, no active infection, inflammation, or significant fibrosis; and presence of available well-vascularized local tissue for transfer (eg, labial fat pad, Singapore flap, preplaced gracilis).

the applicability of this technique, however. Another option for short strictures is the Heineke-Mikulicz approach, in which the strictured segment is incised longitudinally and closed transversely to augment the size of the urethral lumen (**Fig. 5**).[9] Excision and primary anastomosis (EPA), in which the strictured segment is excised and healthy ends spatulated

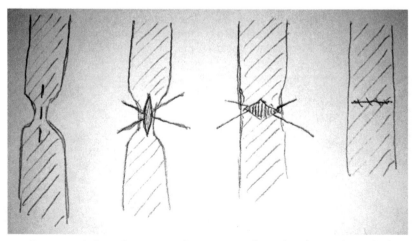

Fig. 5. Diagrammatic representation of nontransecting anastomotic urethroplasty using Heineke-Mikulicz principle: vertical urethrotomy followed by horizontal closure to achieve patent lumen.

and anastomosed, is the gold standard for short urethral strictures in native male urethras (**Fig. 6**).[20] However, the applicability of EPA is notably limited in the transgender patient because of the lack of tissue mobility and good blood supply.[17] The successful use of EPA has been described for short strictures up to 2 to 3 cm long, particularly at the anastomosis when excision of dense scar is required.[9,12] In the largest series of neophallus urethroplasties by Lumen and colleagues,[19] the success of EPA was 57%.

Single-Stage Substitution Techniques

For longer segments of stricture, a flap or graft can be performed in a 1-stage or 2-stage approach. A dorsal inlay approach[21] has been described for 1-stage procedures[19] and skin, bladder mucosa, and buccal mucosa grafts (BMGs) have been used.[17,19] For this approach, a ventral urethrotomy is made to expose the dorsal aspect of the strictured urethra. A vertical incision is made in the dorsal surface of the urethra, and a graft is placed into this dorsal urethrotomy to increase the lumen of the strictured urethra (**Fig. 7**). The BMG has become the graft of choice for urethral reconstruction. It has a pan-laminar vascular plexus ideal for engraftment and a thick nonkeratinized epithelium compatible with a wet environment. It is also readily available and has a hidden harvest site. Given the lack of corpus spongiosum, the vascularity and the coverage of the ventral tissues are unreliable, making the dorsal position of the graft favorable. The urethra is opened ventrally and a dorsal inlay is placed due to better vascularity of the backing tissue on the dorsal aspect. Although in the urethroplasty literature, the dorsal onlay approach with circumferential mobilization is performed in native pendulous urethras, we do not recommend circumferential mobilization of the neourethra, as this would likely result in disruption of the vascular supply. If the vascular supply is tenuous on the recipient site, a fasciocutaneous or muscular flap may be used to support a ventral onlay graft. For strictures in more proximal perineal or neoscrotal locations, overlapping double-face grafts were successfully used by the authors. In addition to the dorsal inlays, ventral BMG onlays were placed to increase the surface of the lumen. Vascularization of the ventral grafts was achieved by rotating the labial fat pad from the neoscrotum (**Fig. 8**), or when available, by "recycling" a gracilis flap brought to the perineum during the original operation (**Fig. 9**).

Staged Techniques

In a 2-stage urethroplasty, the ventral urethrotomy is made through the stricture segment. The existing urethral plate can be augmented with graft material and the lateral edges of the new urethral plate is sutured to the borders of the skin incision. Once the new urethral plate has matured, typically 6 months later, the new augmented urethral plate is tubularized and the neophallus closed. This is the preferred technique for long or refractory strictures.[9] Success rates of 70% were reported by

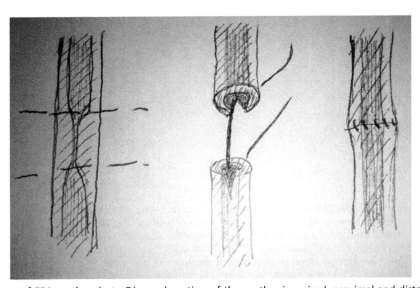

Fig. 6. Diagram of EPA urethroplasty. Diseased portion of the urethra is excised, proximal and distal stumps are spatulated in opposite complementary directions, and the spatulated ends are sutured together to create patent anastomosis.

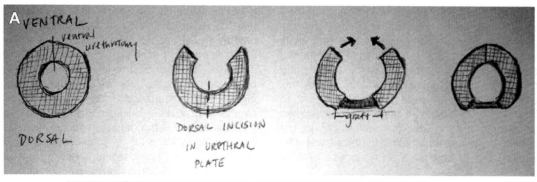

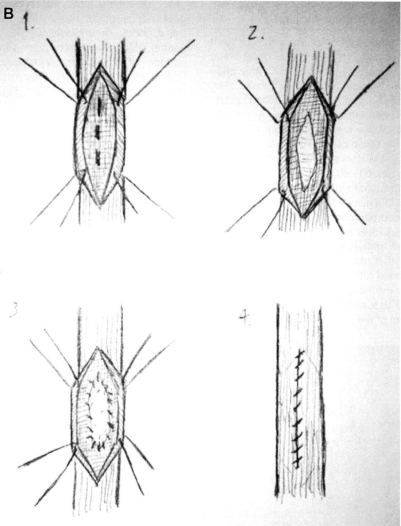

Fig. 7. Diagram of dorsal inlay (Asopa type) urethroplasty: (*A*) cross-section view and (*B*) ventral view of urethral segment. Ventral urethrotomy is created to achieve access to dorsal surface of diseased urethra, dorsal longitudinal incision is made through the narrow portion, appropriate-size BMG is quilted as a dorsal inlay into the defect, and ventral urethrotomy is closed. Ventral urethrotomy (1) is created to achieve access to dorsal surface of diseased urethra, dorsal longitudinal incision is made through the narrow portion (2), appropriate-size BMG is quilted as a dorsal inlay (3) into the defect, and ventral urethrotomy is closed (4).

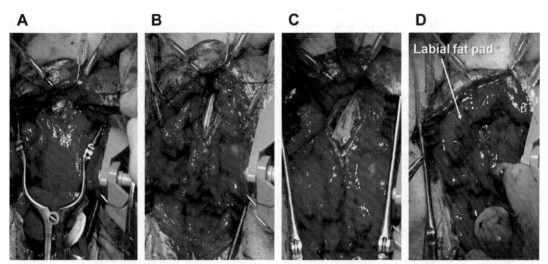

Fig. 8. Example of a single-stage urethroplasty using double-face BMG. (*A*) Dorsal inlay BMG (Asopa type) is completed, (*B*) catheter is placed across the reconstructed portion in preparation for ventral onlay, (*C*) the second buccal graft is tailored for ventral onlay, and (*D*) the ventral graft is secured to the edges of the neourethra in preparation to be quilted to the right labial fad pad.

Lumen and colleagues,[19] the highest among all types of neophallic urethroplasty.

Perineal Urethrostomy

Perineal urethrostomy is also an option if multiple reconstructive efforts fail, or if it is the patient's preference. The segment of fixed urethra can be opened and approximated to the perineum so as to expose the native urethral meatus. This may also be used as a temporary treatment until definitive reconstruction can take place. A combination of several reconstructive approaches may be required for multifocal stricture. Regardless of the approach to urethral reconstruction, stricture recurrence rates after treatments are more than 60%,[9] with many patients requiring repeated interventions.[12]

RESULTS

At our institutions we select the technique of reconstruction based on the patient's new anatomy and condition of the tissues. For example, the retrograde urethrogram in **Fig. 1** demonstrates a patient with a 4-cm urethral stricture of the anastomotic urethra extending proximally into the fixed urethra and distally into the phallic urethra. A stricture of this length cannot be reconstructed by Heineke-Mikulicz or EPA. The urethra was opened, and a BMG was placed dorsally (**Fig. 10**A). The ventral urethra was covered with the BMG, and a fasciocutaneous flap was sutured to the graft (**Fig. 10**B). The fasciocutaneous flap was incorporated into the neophallus, and the patient was able to void well after surgery (**Fig. 10**C).

In another patient with a stricture of the anastomotic urethra and phallic urethra, the obstruction resulted in a fistula communicating with a persistent vaginal cavity (**Fig. 11**A). The cavity was resected using a transabdominal robotic-assisted laparoscopic approach (**Fig. 11**B). As the patient had a long urethral stenosis, a first-stage urethroplasty using BMG was performed (**Fig. 11**C). This patient is currently awaiting second-stage reconstruction.

Patients after metoidioplasty may present with isolated distal neourethral stricture or combination of stricture and fistulization into a remnant vaginal cavity. In the first such example, the patient demonstrated significant neourethral scarring and required a 2-stage BMG augmented reconstruction (**Fig. 12**). Another patient presented with a combination of neourethral stricture and recurrent vaginal cavity communicating with ventral urethral fistula. This patient already had gracilis flap placed into the perineum at the time of primary surgery in hopes of preventing urethrocutaneous fistula. For this patient, 1-stage reconstruction was offered that involved the following steps: (1) dissection and preservation of the gracilis; (2) excision and obliteration of the vaginal cavity; (3) splitting of the gracilis into 2 "tails," one of which was repurposed for vaginal cavity obliteration, and the other tail used as a bed for ventral BMG support; (4) dorsal BMG inlay for urethral stricture; and (5) ventral onlay BMG supported by the second "tail" of the recycled gracilis (see **Fig. 9**).

Although many patients would prefer to void while standing, the patient may elect to undergo

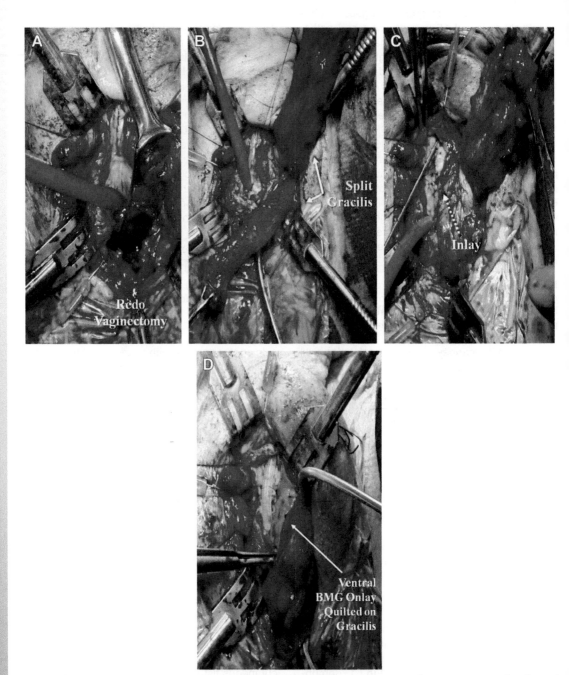

Fig. 9. Example of single-stage double-face urethroplasty for simultaneous repair of persistent vaginal cavity and long neourethral stricture in a patient with previously rotated gracilis flap. (*A*) Redo vaginectomy is performed, gracilis is preserved and retracted away, and neourethra is opened ventrally. (*B*) The gracilis is divided into 2 segments. One segment is used to support the BMG, and the other segment is used to obliterate a persistent vaginal cavity. (*C*) BMG dorsal inlay (Asopa type). (*D*) Creation of ventral hemiplate by quilting BMG onto gracilis and anastomosis of this composite to the edges of the native urethra.

a perineal urethrostomy as a temporizing measure (**Fig. 13**). Further reconstruction to allow the patient to stand to void may be performed in the future.

PROBLEMS AND COMPLICATIONS

There are several challenges to urinary reconstruction after phalloplasty in the female-to-male transgendered patient.[9] There is no native corpus

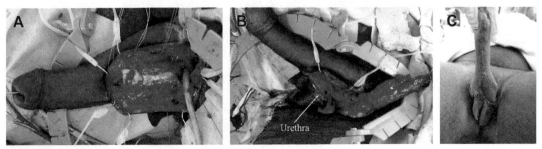

Fig. 10. (*A*) urethra is opened through a ventral urethrotomy, buccal graft is placed and secured dorsaly. (*B*) ventral urethral plate is created using rotated fasciocutaneous flap anastomosed side-to-side to the dorsal BMG and end-to-end to the spatulated ends of the neo-urethra. (*C*) final appearance of the reconstructed neophallus.

spongiosum to cover the urethral reconstruction. Preputial and penile skin flaps commonly used in standard penile urethral reconstruction are not available in these individuals and therefore extragenital grafts and flaps must be used.[17] There may be dense scar tissue present after the phalloplasty. Furthermore, the neophallus is made up of skin, fat, and fascia, which may not be the ideal vascularized graft recipient site.[12]

Even after successful reconstruction, urinary incontinence is prevalent in the female-to-male transgendered population, due to trapping of urine in the fixed and phallic parts of the urethra.[22] The long-term effect of a neourethra on bladder function is unknown, and given the high propensity for recurrence of strictures and urinary fistulae, lifelong urologic follow-up is of paramount importance.[18]

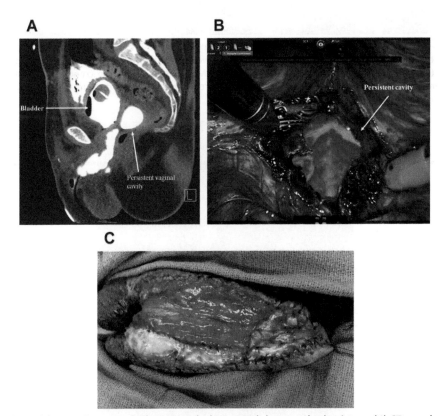

Fig. 11. Patient with a persistent vaginal cavity and a long pendulous urethral stricture. (*A*) CT scan showing large persistent fluid-filled cavity inferior to the bladder. (*B*) Robotic-assisted laparoscopic redo vaginectomy. (*C*) Removed vaginal epithelium is used as a graft for a first-stage urethroplasty.

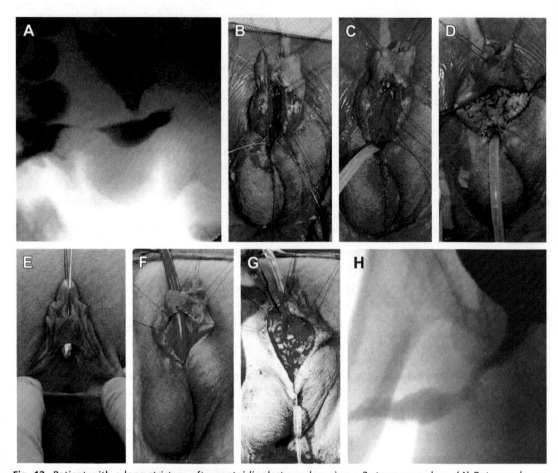

Fig. 12. Patient with a long stricture after metoidioplasty undergoing a 2-stage procedure. (*A*) Retrograde urethrogram showing the stricture. (*B*) Ventral urethrotomy over the stricture segment sparing the neoglans and neomeatus. (*C*) Removal of diseased segment. (*D*) Dorsal BMG graft is quilted to create future urethral plate. (*E–G*) Appearance of the urethral plate 6 months later before the second stage (tubularization). (*H*) Voiding cystourethrogram 4 weeks after the operation.

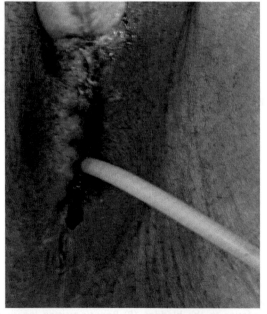

Fig. 13. Example of perineal urethrostomy in a patient with long neourethral stricture who preferred to avoid multistage reconstruction.

REFERENCES

1. Collin L, Reisner SL, Tangpricha V, et al. Prevalence of transgender depends on the "case" definition: a systematic review. J Sex Med 2016;13(4):613–26.
2. Horbach SER, Bouman M-B, Smit JM, et al. Outcome of vaginoplasty in male-to-female transgenders: a systematic review of surgical techniques. J Sex Med 2015;12(6):1499–512.
3. van der Sluis WB, Bouman MB, Buncamper ME, et al. Clinical characteristics and management of neovaginal fistulas after vaginoplasty in transgender women. Obstet Gynecol 2016;127(6):1118–26.
4. Dubin BJ, Sato RM, Laub DR. Results of phalloplasty. Plast Reconstr Surg 1979;64(2):163–70.
5. Puckett CL, Montie JE. Construction of male genitalia in the transsexual, using a tubed groin flap for the penis and a hydraulic inflation device. Plast Reconstr Surg 1978;61(4):523–30.
6. Hage JJ, Bloem JJ. Review of the literature on construction of a neourethra in female-to-male transsexuals. Ann Plast Surg 1993;30(3):278–86.
7. Hage JJ, Bout CA, Bloem JJ, et al. Phalloplasty in female-to-male transsexuals: what do our patients ask for? Ann Plast Surg 1993;30(4):323–6.
8. Perovic SV, Djordjevic ML. Metoidioplasty: a variant of phalloplasty in female transsexuals. BJU Int 2003;92(9):981–5.
9. Lumen N, Monstrey S, Goessaert AS, et al. Urethroplasty for strictures after phallic reconstruction: a single-institution experience. Eur Urol 2011;60(1):150–8.
10. Rashid M, Tamimy MS. Phalloplasty: the dream and the reality. Indian J Plast Surg 2013;46(2):283–93.
11. Rashid M, Sarwar SR. Avulsion injuries of the male external genitalia: classification and reconstruction with the customised radial forearm free flap. Br J Plast Surg 2005;58(5):585–92.
12. Rohrmann D, Jakse G. Urethroplasty in female-to-male transsexuals. Eur Urol 2003;44(5):611–4.
13. Leriche A, Timsit MO, Morel-Journel N, et al. Long-term outcome of forearm flee-flap phalloplasty in the treatment of transsexualism. BJU Int 2008;101(10):1297–300.
14. Kim SK, Moon JB, Heo J, et al. A new method of urethroplasty for prevention of fistula in female-to-male gender reassignment surgery. Ann Plast Surg 2010;64(6):759–64.
15. Blaschke E, Bales GT, Thomas S. Postoperative imaging of phalloplasties and their complications. Am J Roentgenol 2014;203(2):323–8.
16. Fang RH, Kao YS, Ma S, et al. Phalloplasty in female-to-male transsexuals using free radial osteocutaneous flap: a series of 22 cases. Br J Plast Surg 1999;52(3):217–22.
17. Levine LA, Elterman L. Urethroplasty following total phallic reconstruction. J Urol 1998;160(2):378–82.
18. Monstrey SJ, Ceulemans P, Hoebeke P. Sex reassignment surgery in the female-to-male transsexual. Semin Plast Surg 2011;25(3):229–44.
19. Lumen N, Oosterlinck W, Decaestecker K, et al. Endoscopic incision of short (<3 cm) urethral strictures after phallic reconstruction. J Endourol 2009;23(8):1329–32.
20. Morey AF, McAninch JW. When and how to use buccal mucosal grafts in adult bulbar urethroplasty. Urology 1996;48(2):194–8.
21. Asopa HS, Garg M, Singhal GG, et al. Dorsal free graft urethroplasty for urethral stricture by ventral sagittal urethrotomy approach. Urology 2001;58(5):657–9.
22. Hoebeke P, Selvaggi G, Ceulemans P, et al. Impact of sex reassignment surgery on lower urinary tract function. Eur Urol 2005;47(3):398–402.

Use of Alternative Techniques and Grafts in Urethroplasty

Brendan Michael Browne, MD, MS, Alex J. Vanni, MD*

KEYWORDS

- Urethral stricture • Urethroplasty • Urethral reconstruction • Injectable antifibrotic treatment
- Augmentation urethroplasty • Lingual mucosa graft • Colonic mucosa graft
- Tissue-engineered graft

KEY POINTS

- Injectable antifibrotic agents may improve rates of recurrence compared with direct vision internal urethrotomy for short urethral strictures.
- Lingual mucosa has similar physiologic and anatomic characteristics to buccal mucosa with promising outcomes from initial clinical trials.
- Colonic mucosa can be harvested in a minimally invasive fashion, thereby increasing its potential use as a graft in complex cases of urethral reconstruction.
- Acellular matrices and tissue-engineered grafts have begun small clinical trials and may eventually provide an off-the-shelf option for urethral reconstruction.

INTRODUCTION

The repair of urethral stricture is approached with multiple different techniques, ranging from endoscopic incision to graft placement for open reconstruction, in an attempt to open and maintain a normal urethral lumen. All causes of stricture, including trauma, iatrogenic injury, lichen sclerosus, or prior urethral surgery, have the potential to form long, complex strictures that necessitate extensive reconstruction. Treatment selection ultimately depends on the cause of the stricture, location, length, and the surgeon's preference and experience level. Shorter strictures are amenable to endoscopic treatment or excision and anastomosis, whereas longer defects require augmentation with oral mucosa grafts or fasciocutaneous flaps. However, clinical scenarios exist whereby the typical buccal mucosa graft or fasciocutaneous flap is insufficient for urethral reconstruction.

Current practice of urethral reconstruction places a premium on buccal mucosa grafts, but additional grafts are available to use as an alternative or adjunct in complex cases, particularly panurethral strictures, recurrent strictures when buccal mucosa has been previously harvested, or in patients in whom retrieval of oral mucosa in contraindicated. Buccal mucosa has enjoyed such success that many of the original grafts for urethroplasty, such as extragenital skin, have fallen out of favor. Despite the decreased utilization of skin grafts, the principles of this technique should be continually revisited for inspiration and innovation toward new approaches. Furthermore, tissue engineering and stem cell therapies are promising opportunities to provide off-the-shelf grafts that would preclude the invasiveness and morbidity of tissue harvest for urethral reconstruction.

Disclosure Statement: The authors have no disclosures to identify.
Department of Urology, Lahey Hospital and Medical Center, 41 Mall Road, Burlington, MA 01805, USA
* Corresponding author.
E-mail address: Alex.J.Vanni@Lahey.org

INJECTABLES

Although open urethroplasty is the gold standard for treatment of anterior urethral strictures, endoscopic management offers options that are less invasive and can be effective in highly selected patients. Current endoscopic treatments achieve inferior outcomes to open repair,[1,2] so any improvements in endoscopic platforms that could open this treatment to a broader patient base are intriguing. In addition to stricture incision, multiple antifibrotic medications have been used in attempt to reduce scar formation and inhibit tissue contraction.

Combination of the traditional direct vision internal urethrotomy (DVIU) with topical application or injection of an antiproliferative agent has been evaluated for minimally invasive stricture treatment. Antifibrotic agents, including steroids (triamcinolone), mitomycin C (MMC), and hyaluronidase, have all been used to reduce stricture recurrence. The antifibrotic and anticollagen properties of steroids are well documented, and injectable forms are used in treatment of various fibrosis-induced pathologies. MMC has been shown to inhibit cellular proliferation and collagen deposition during scar formation in both in vitro and animal studies.[3,4] Additionally, MMC has been used clinically for pathologies ranging from nasolacrimal duct obstruction and to vaginal and anal stenosis.[5–10] Hyaluronidase also possesses antifibrotic properties and has shown benefits in treatment of pulmonary fibrosis, hypertrophic scars, and keloids. Its function is achieved by suppression of fibroblast synthesis of collagen and glycosaminoglycan, which are necessary building blocks for scar formation.[11] Although these agents have a clear theoretic and clinical role for scar management, there are few high-quality studies examining the efficacy of injected antiproliferative agents for anterior urethral strictures.

Triamcinolone has the most published experience, with trials of injected and catheter-coated topical administration dating back to the 1960s.[12] Urethrotomy followed by triamcinolone injection has been shown to be safe and moderately effective. Two small randomized controlled trials evaluated the effect of triamcinolone following urethrotomy for short bulbar strictures (<1.5 cm).[13,14] Mazdak and colleagues[14] reported stricture recurrence in 21.7% of the triamcinolone group versus 50.0% of the control cohort at a follow-up of 14 months. Meanwhile, Tavakkoli and colleagues[13] reported a lower number of recurrences in the triamcinolone group, but this finding was not statistically significant. A meta-analysis of 8 studies covering 203 patients showed no benefit for catheter-introduced steroids following DVIU, but steroid injection prolonged the time to stricture recurrence.[15]

MMC is also gaining attention as an injectable antiscar agent. The first randomized controlled trial to study MMC following DVIU in short bulbar urethral strictures found a recurrence rate of 10% in the MMC group compared with 50% for DVIU alone. Of note, this study only included 40 total patients and had relatively short follow-up (range 6–24 months).[16] These findings were supported by a recent randomized controlled trial that compared DVIU with MMC to DVIU alone in 151 patients with traumatic anterior urethral strictures measuring up to 2 cm in length. The patients were then followed with retrograde urethrography at 3-month intervals for 18 months. Stricture recurrence was identified in 14% of the MMC group compared with 37% of the control group ($P = .002$), and the time to recurrence was 3 months longer in patients treated with MMC ($P = .002$).[17]

Although hyaluronic acid has shown antifibrotic effects in animal models,[18] there has been minimal experience in humans. One randomized controlled trial examined the effect of hyaluronic acid and carboxymethylcellulose urethral instillation after DVIU. The experimental group had a significantly lower recurrence rate than controls (9.4% vs 22.9%).[19] These patients were only followed for 6 months, and more data are needed before definitive conclusions can be made for this treatment.

Injection of all 3 drugs simultaneously has also been proposed to reduce stricture recurrence following DVIU. A mixture of 40 mg triamcinolone, 2 mg MMC, and 3000 units of hyaluronic acid were injected into 103 patients with bulbar and penile urethral strictures with no control group. Following one procedure, strictures recurred in 19.4% of cases at a median follow-up of 14 months (range 3–18 months).[20] However, the validity of this study is in question as the lack of a control group precludes any definitive evaluation of this technique.

Other injectable therapies for anterior urethral stricture are in the nascent phase of investigation. Medications that have proven safe and effective for other urologic pathologies are being trialed for urethral stricture. Botox injection following DVIU was reported with modest improvement in short follow-up on 3 patients.[21] Additionally, collagenase *Clostridium histolyticum*, an injectable therapy for dissolution of Peyronie disease plaques, showed reduction in collagen expression and fibrosis in a rat model of urethral stricture.[22] Animal models have also tested the treatment of urethral strictures with topical bevacizumab, 5-fluorouracil, and halofuginone with promising early results.[23,24]

Antifibrotic injectables have been steadily growing since their introduction almost 50 years ago, with new agents being continually explored. More rigorous clinical trials to evaluate long-term outcomes and with more clearly defined stricture recurrence criteria are needed to confirm results compared with traditional treatments and to identify optimal patients for endoscopic management. Once the role for injectable treatments is more clearly delineated, their widespread use could allow more patients to avoid the morbidity of open reconstruction.

ALTERNATIVE GRAFTS

Placement of tissue grafts to enlarge or replace the urethral lumen is a long-standing practice for urethral reconstruction. Skin grafts or flaps were some of the original tissues used for urethral reconstruction, but several new sources of graft material have arisen over the past decades. Options include lingual mucosal grafts, bladder epithelium, colonic mucosa, and tissue-engineered grafts, which can all be used for urethroplasty in complex cases.

Genital and Extragenital Skin

Urethral reconstruction with penile skin was first described by Presman and Greenfield[25] in 1953 and gained prominence with preputial skin grafting for hypospadias repair.[25,26] Penile skin can be deployed as either a flap or graft, which achieve similar efficacy for urethral reconstruction.[27,28] However, there is significantly less morbidity with the use of grafts, namely, reduced penile skin necrosis and penile torsion.[29,30] Harvesting well-vascularized penile skin flaps is technically challenging; thus, full-thickness skin grafts have gained the favor of reconstructive surgeons. Genital and extragenital skin grafts are less common in the era of buccal mucosa urethroplasty, but they still play a key role in urethral reconstruction. Although skin grafts should be avoided in patients with lichen sclerosus, they can provide long tissue segments when buccal mucosa has been damaged by tobacco, radiation, or oral leukoplakia or for cases whereby oral mucosa has previously been harvested. Penile skin has the benefits of being elastic, well-vascularized tissue that is devoid of hair. Graft harvest from the penis is relatively straightforward and results in minimal morbidity. A meta-analysis comparing penile skin versus buccal mucosa for urethral reconstruction reported improved outcomes in the buccal mucosa group, achieving 85.9% success compared with 81.8% for penile skin graft ($P = .01$).[31] However, it should be noted that the penile skin graft group had an average

follow-up almost 2 years longer (64 months skin versus 42 months) and longer stricture length (6.2 cm versus 4.6 cm) than the buccal mucosa cohort. To examine the long-term outcomes of oral mucosa or penile skin graft urethroplasty, Barbagli and colleagues[32] recently published a series of 359 patients followed for a minimum of 6 years. They found a 59.7% success rate for penile skin grafts versus 77.7% for oral mucosa grafts. Furthermore, penile skin grafts were a significant predictor of graft failure on multivariate analysis, even when adjusting for age, stricture length, cause, and previous treatments.[32]

Postauricular skin can serve as an alternative full-thickness graft when oral mucosa and genital skin are inadequate or unavailable for urethroplasty. The best tissue for harvest is located along the lower half of the mastoid and posterior to the tragus, which can yield a graft measuring up to 8 cm from each side. Manoj and colleagues[33] performed anterior urethroplasty on 35 patients and achieved an 89% success rate after 21 months of follow-up. They reported no donor-site complications. For 2-stage hypospadias repairs, Nitkunan and colleagues[34] reported a 97% success rate for graft uptake, with the single failure resulting from keloid formation on the graft, identifying a complication unique to skin grafts. The donor site of this graft is easily visible, and when harvesting this tissue every attempt should be made to maximize cosmesis.

Abdominal skin can also provide full-thickness skin graft for urethral reconstruction. Optimal abdominal skin is located along the flank and lower abdomen, where there are fewer hair follicles. This graft also should be used for patients who have no signs of lichen sclerosus and who lack adequate oral mucosa. It has proven useful as an adjunct to buccal mucosa, as exemplified by Chen and colleagues[35] who combined a dorsal full-thickness abdominal skin graft with ventral buccal mucosa graft for complex bulbar urethral strictures. For patients with strictures greater than 6 cm, they achieved a 100% success rate. In contrast, Liu and colleagues[36] reported on a group of 26 men treated with abdominal wall skin grafts versus 213 treated with other grafts over a median of 59 months of follow-up. The recurrence rate was 53% for the abdominal wall grafts compared with 24% for the others. Multivariate analysis of this cohort identified lichen sclerosus and prior urethroplasty as predictors of recurrence. Although graft type did not predict recurrence in this study, the use of abdominal skin in patients with lichen sclerosus likely influences the poor outcomes observed in these patients.[36] Further studies are needed to elucidate the role of abdominal skin grafts as stand-alone or combination grafts in urethral reconstruction.

Although the original skin grafts were harvested as full-thickness sections, split-thickness skin grafts with mesh support offer a modified approach to skin grafting for augmentation urethroplasty. Schreiter and Noll[37] promoted 2-stage urethral reconstruction with these grafts for patients with long complex strictures and severe spongiofibrosis. Long-term success has been reported as 79% at 6.5 years, even in highly complex strictures.[38] Furthermore, use of meshed grafts cause minimal complications, reporting erectile dysfunction in 4% and penile curvature in 9% of patients following 2-stage urethroplasty.[39] In the current era of buccal mucosa urethroplasty, skin grafts account for a small percentage of overall reconstruction; but they can prove useful in place of or in conjunction with oral grafts for the most complex urethral strictures.

Lingual Grafts

The biological qualities of oral mucosa, including adaptation to a fluid environment and relative resistance to lichen sclerosus, make it ideal for augmentation urethroplasty.[40,41] Clinical data regarding lingual mucosa grafts are not as extensive as for buccal mucosa, but the similar anatomic and physiologic characteristics make lingual grafts similarly appealing. Both grafts display a thick epithelial layer with thin lamina propria and a robust, pan-laminar vascular bed, which facilitates graft take and minimizes contracture. Because of the similar architecture, lingual mucosa can serve as an ideal substitute when buccal mucosa has already been harvested or as an additional graft for repair of long defects.[42]

Harvest of lingual grafts is equally straightforward as buccal mucosa. The mucosa is readily accessible, can produce 2 grafts from 7 to 16 cm long, and leaves no visible scar at the harvest site. The lateral and ventral surfaces of the tongue can be used as individual grafts or a combination of both sections when larger segments are required.[42–44] While procuring the graft, the appropriate plane of dissection is between the mucosa and submucosal fat. Identifying the Wharton duct and the lingual nerve as well as the floor of the mouth is critical, as scarring in these sites will reduce tongue mobility postoperatively.[43] Before use, the fibrovascular tissue underlying the graft should be manually removed to help with graft take. Closure of the harvest site with an absorbable suture achieves optimal healing.

Urethral reconstruction with lingual grafts can be performed in the same manner as any urethral reconstruction; with both one-stage (dorsal onlay, dorsal inlay, ventral onlay) or 2-stage approaches a viable option. The studies examining lingual mucosal grafting for urethral reconstruction are summarized in **Table 1**.[42–48] Success rates ranged from 79% to 96%, but most of these studies encompass small numbers with short follow-up. Abdelhameed and colleagues[47] measured the long-term outcomes of lingual grafts in 23 patients, showing 87% freedom from restricture at 66 months of follow-up. Of note, the stricture cause and surgical techniques were heterogeneous in these studies; longer follow-up is needed to determine the long-term outcomes of this graft. Four groups undertook randomized comparisons of lingual versus buccal grafts, shown in **Table 2**.[49–52] Three of them showed comparable success rates between buccal and lingual grafts, but the largest comparison completed by Chauhan and colleagues[50] found lingual grafts superior to buccal grafts with 80% and 69% success, respectively, at 25 months.

Lingual mucosa grafts can be especially useful in patients with lichen sclerosus, who are prone to long and recurrent strictures. Some panurethral strictures are longer than the available buccal mucosa is able to repair, whereas others will have recurrence of their stricture after bilateral buccal graft urethroplasty and need subsequent reconstruction. Das and colleagues[45] reported short-term outcomes on 30 patients undergoing lingual mucosa urethroplasty, of whom 18 had lichen sclerosus. Their overall success rate was 83.3% with an average follow-up of 9 months. Furthermore, Xu and colleagues[53] analyzed one-stage lingual mucosa grafting, specifically in patients with lichen sclerosus–induced strictures averaging 12.5 cm in length. They also reported positive results, achieving 90.9% success rate in 22 patients with lichen sclerosus with 38 months of follow-up.

Although lingual mucosa has notable positive characteristics, its use does may cause appreciable patient morbidity. Several studies have specifically investigated postoperative pain and disability at the harvest site. Pain in the mouth was mostly limited to the first 1 to 2 days, and all patients were pain free by postoperative day 6. As would be expected, bilateral lingual graft harvest caused a slight increase in postoperative pain.[54,55] Also of note, harvest of lingual grafts longer than 7 cm or bilateral grafts was more likely to cause long-term speech changes.[49] Lumen and colleagues[51] compared the postoperative morbidity of lingual versus buccal graft harvest and found that the functional impairment (ie, difficulty eating or speaking) were higher in lingual

Table 1
Clinical studies of lingual mucosa grafts

Author	No. of Patients	Average Follow-up (mo)	Stricture Length	Surgical Technique	Success (Definition of Success)	Complications
Simonato et al,[42] 2008	29	17.7	3.6 cm	1- or 2-Stage onlay	79.3%, No repeat intervention	None reported
Barbagli et al,[43] 2008	10	5	4.5 cm	Dorsal inlay or ventral onlay	90%, No repeat intervention	Urethrocutaneous fistula (10%)
Xu et al,[44] 2010	92	17 (3–33)	6.5 cm (2.5–18.0)	50 Dorsal onlay, 42 tubularized substitute	96%, No stricture recurrence or need for procedure	Urethrocutaneous fistula (4%)
Das et al,[45] 2009	30	9 (4–12)	10.2 cm (3.7–16.0)	Dorsal onlay	83.3%, No repeat instrumentation and peak flow >15 mL/s	Wound infection (7%), extravasation (17%), temporary chordae (3%)
Sharma et al,[46] 2010	15	12	2.45 cm	Dorsal onlay	93%, No postoperative instrumentation	None reported
Abdelhameed et al,[47] 2015	23	66 (60–72)	4.6 cm	15 Dorsal onlay, 8 ventral onlay	87%, No restriction on RUG, no postoperative instrumentation	Wound infection (17%), extravasation (4%), oral numbness (39%), postvoid dribbling (13%)
Li et al,[48] 2016	56	34.7 (10–58)	5.6 cm ±1.6	42 Ventral onlay, 14 Snodgrass inlay	78.6%, No restriction or fistula	Urethrocutaneous fistula (12.5%), neourethral stricture (9%), meatal stenosis (4%)

Abbreviation: RUG, retrograde urethrogram.

Table 2
Clinical trials of buccal mucosa versus lingual mucosa grafts

Author	No. BMG	No. LMG	Avg F/U (Range)	Avg Stricture Length (Range)	Success (Definition of Success)
Sharma et al,[49] 2013	15	15	14.5 mo	8.1 cm	86.7% BMG vs 93.3% LMG No stricture on urethroscopy, flow >15 mL/s
Chauhan et al,[50] 2016	52	50	25.0 mo	6.5 cm (3.2–13.5)	69.2% BMG vs 80.0% LMG No obstructive voiding or instrumentation
Lumen et al,[51] 2016	29	29	30.0 mo (17–43)	5.0 cm (1–18)	82.8% BMG vs 89.7% LMG No stricture, fistula, or urethral manipulation
Maarouf et al,[52] 2013	23	21	20.8 mo (12–24)	6.8 cm	78.2% BMG vs 76.1% LMG No postoperative procedure

Abbreviations: Avg, average; BMG, buccal mucosa graft; F/U, follow-up; LMG, lingual mucosa graft.

grafts through the first 2 weeks postoperatively, but there was no difference in long-term sequelae between the two groups. Graft-site morbidity for studies comparing buccal and lingual mucosa grafts is compiled in **Table 3**.[49–52]

Lingual grafts provide a high-quality alternative for buccal mucosa for augmentation urethroplasty in patients who have long defects or recurrent strictures. The lingual mucosal surface is easily accessible and sufficiently isolated from buccal mucosa to not be damaged by prior buccal mucosa harvest. Early clinical data show urethral reconstruction with lingual mucosa to achieve equal success to buccal mucosa, but larger studies with longer follow-up are needed to confirm these findings. Also, harvest-site morbidity should be considered when treating long strictures, as there is no established safe graft length and larger grafts may cause long-term speech and eating disabilities.

Bladder Mucosa

Bladder mucosa may be harvested to create a graft that has most commonly been used for hypospadias repair. The graft is rarely used because of the invasive harvest, which is accomplished by an open bladder dissection, in addition to frequent stricture recurrence. Meatal problems are reported in 68% of patients, and repeat procedures are required in two-thirds of patients to achieve successful outcomes.[56]

Table 3
Comparison of oral graft harvest site morbidity

	Early Postoperative (<1 wk)		Intermediate Postoperative (3–6 mo)		Late Postoperative (1 y)	
	Buccal Graft	Lingual Graft	Buccal Graft	Lingual Graft	Buccal Graft	Lingual Graft
Bleeding	6/67 (9%)	9/65 (14%)	0/67 (0%)	0/65 (0%)	0/67 (0%)	0/65 (0%)
Oral pain	72/104 (69%)	40/100 (40%)	1/81 (1%)	0/79 (0%)	0/67 (0%)	0/65 (0%)
Mouth tightness	68/90 (76%)	23/86 (27%)	13/94 (14%)	2/94 (2%)	0/67 (0%)	0/65 (0%)
Speech difficulty	50/119 (42%)	84/115 (73%)	12/94 (13%)	14/94 (15%)	0/67 (0%)	4/65 (6%)
Altered sensation	88/119 (74%)	52/115 (45%)	25/117 (21%)	12/115 (10%)	2/67 (3%)	0/65 (0%)
Difficulty chewing	54/96 (56%)	57/94 (61%)	22/94 (23%)	12/94 (13%)	0/67 (0%)	0/65 (0%)
Reduced tongue protrusion	5/38 (13%)	36/36 (100%)	0/15 (0%)	3/15 (20%)	0/67 (0%)	2/65 (3%)

Colonic Mucosa

Colonic mucosa has recently gained attention as a tissue source for long segment urethral strictures. Xu and colleagues[57] first reported the use of tubularized colonic mucosa for urethroplasty in 2004. When the same group examined the outcomes for 36 patients after 4.5 years of follow-up, they found an 85.7% success rate for strictures averaging 15.1 cm in length.[58] The clear downside to this graft is that all of these patients required sigmoid resection to harvest the graft material, imposing significant morbidity. For salvage urethroplasty at the authors' institution, they have begun using a transanal endoscopic microsurgical technique (TEM) (**Figs. 1–4**) to harvest colonic mucosa without a bowel resection. The TEM technique was originally designed by colorectal surgeons for minimally invasive access to rectal tumors or polyps. The TEM technique is able to reach tissue 20 cm above the anal verge and, thus, is ideally suited for harvest of long graft segments. The authors have published this approach on 4 patients with no complications from the colonic mucosa harvest.[59] After 18 months of follow-up (range 12–28 months), 3 out of 4 patients have had successful urethral reconstruction, with the remaining patient demonstrating stricture recurrence treated with urethral dilation. The average stricture length was 13.5 cm (range

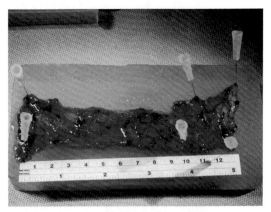

Fig. 2. Colonic mucosa graft before cleaning.

10–21 cm), further demonstrating the potential for harvest of large tissue segments via TEM visualization. Importantly, no patients reported change in bowel function. Larger patient numbers and long-term outcomes will be needed to show what role colonic mucosa may play for salvage urethroplasty.

Acellular Matrix/Tissue Engineering

Tissue engineering is an emerging frontier of urethral reconstruction and holds substantial promise for developing off-the-shelf graft material. Developing platforms that generate large quantities of graft material but do not require harvest of full-thickness skin or mucosa grafts would markedly reduce the morbidity of augmentation urethroplasty. Cell culture techniques are capable of replicating urothelial cells (UCs) and smooth muscle cells (SMCs) into tissue sheets large enough to replace the native urethra,[60] but these constructs have proven too vulnerable to withstand surgical handling and suturing.[61] To overcome the mechanical stresses of surgical manipulation and

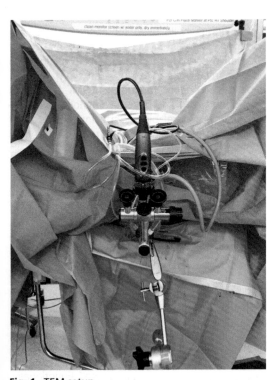

Fig. 1. TEM setup.

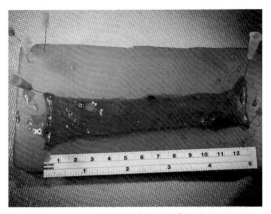

Fig. 3. Colonic mucosa graft ready for placement.

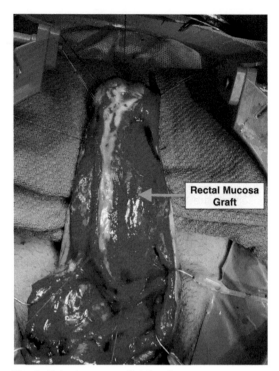

Rectal Mucosa
Graft

Fig. 4. Colonic mucosa dorsal onlay.

transurethral urine flow, biomolecular scaffolds (or matrices) have been developed to provide strength and shape to urethral grafts.

Two main approaches to scaffold construction are used: (1) biological decellularized tissue, including dermis, urinary bladder, or small intestine submucosa (SIS), or (2) synthetic polymers, including polyglycolic acid (PGA), poly-L-lactide-co-ε-caprolactone, and many others.[61] Biological matrices are often harvested from human cadaveric or porcine sources. The tissues are subsequently treated with mechanical, chemical or enzymatic processes to remove cellular components, leaving native collagen and extracellular matrix (ECM) proteins intact. In contrast, synthetic matrices are made via of molding, dipping or electrospinning of polymers.[62] These synthetic constructs have increased mechanical strength relative to biologicals[63] and can be built with a large variety of pore sizes, polymer orientations, and surface properties.

Within both categories of scaffolds, grafts exist that are purely acellular constructs, whereas others are seeded with autologous cells obtained from tissue biopsy, voided urine, or other sources. Cell-seeded matrices have the benefit of cellular proliferation across the entire surface, in addition to ingrowth of adjacent urothelium from the graft edges. Complete reepithelialization of the graft is crucial to a successful outcome, as exposed areas will rapidly form scar tissue.[64] Acellular matrix grafts are successful for onlay grafting or short segment tubularized grafting, but poor native tissue ingrowth is seen in tubularized segments of 1 cm or greater.[64–66] Meanwhile, in rabbit models, cell-seeded tubularized grafts achieved full epithelialization and maintained patency for lengths of 3 cm at 6 months, compared with acellular grafts that all strictured down within the first month.[67]

Cell seeding does show evident benefits; however, the process of adhering cells to a matrix increases the complexity to graft production. Although synthetic scaffolds have superior mechanical strength, biological scaffolds are traditionally more conducive to cell attachment.[68] Improvements in cell adhesion, differentiation, and proliferation on synthetic scaffolds have been achieved with surface adsorption of collagen and other ECM proteins[68–71] to the point that some coated synthetic grafts now show equivalent or improved adhesion and proliferation of UC compared with SIS biological grafts.[72] Additionally, new techniques have used coculture of UC and SMC to more accurately mimic native anatomy. Studies have shown that coseeding of UC and SMC improved cellular proliferation when compared with either cell type alone.[73,74] This synergy is likely due to paracrine cell signaling that enhances cell growth. However, this finding has only been documented for biological grafts, with no studies evaluating combined seeding on synthetic grafts.

Autologous cells used for seeding grafts are commonly harvested via bladder biopsy,[75] but alternative sources of cells are being explored to obviate invasive harvest of urothelium. Tissue-engineered buccal mucosa (TEBM) has been developed to expand buccal keratinocytes and fibroblasts from oral biopsy specimens and seed these cells onto acellular dermal matrix for urethral grafting.[76] Additionally, undifferentiated stem cells have attracted attention for this utility. Embryonic stem cells (ESCs) have been successfully differentiated into UC[77] and seeded onto SIS scaffolds for repair of rat bladders.[78] Because of the significant regulatory and ethical issues attached to ESCs, other sources of adult stem cells (ASCs) have been pursued. ASCs collected from bone marrow,[79] voided urine,[80] and adipose tissue[81] have been seeded onto matrix grafts and implanted into rabbit urethras showing improved proliferation and differentiation compared with acellular grafts. ASCs show promise as a pluripotent source of UC and SMCs without the regulatory and ethical complications of ESCs, but there still remain concerns over possible malignant transformation of ASCs.[82] The utilization of stem cells in

Table 4
Clinical trials of tissue-engineered grafts

Author	No. of Patients	Graft Type	Cell Seeding	Avg F/U (mo)	Technique	Success (Definition of Success)
Le Roux,[65] 2005	9	Porcine SIS	None	24	Endoscopic	25%, No stricture on urethroscopy
Donkov et al,[83] 2006	9	SIS	None	18	Dorsal onlay	89%, No stricture on urethroscopy
Hauser et al,[84] 2006	5	SIS	None	12 (3–17)	Ventral onlay	20%, No stricture on urethroscopy
Fiala et al,[85] 2007	50	SIS	None	31.2	Onlay	80%, No stricture on RUG
Farahat et al,[86] 2009	10	SIS	None	12–18	Endoscopic DVIU and balloon graft deployment	80%, Normal uroflow and normal RUG
Mantovani et al,[87] 2002	5	SIS	None	6	Dorsal onlay	100%, Normal RUG, asymptomatic, no repeat procedures
Mantovani et al,[88] 2011	40	SIS	None	120	Ventral onlay	100%
Palminteri et al,[89] 2012	25	SIS	None	71	Onlay	76% Overall; ≤4 cm 86%, >4 cm 0%, no repeat instrumentation
Orabi et al,[90] 2013	12	SIS	None	23 (6–36)	Onlay	50% No repeat instrumentation
el-Kassaby et al,[91] 2008	9	Human bladder ACMG	None	25 (18–36)	Ventral onlay	89%, No repeat instrumentation
el-Kassaby et al,[92] 2003	28	Human bladder ACMG	None	37 (36–48)	Ventral onlay	86%, No repeat instrumentation
Fossum et al,[93] 2012	6	Acellular dermis	UCs	86 (72–100)	Onlay	83%, No repeat instrumentation
Raya-Rivera et al,[94] 2011	5	PGA	Human UCs + SMCs	71 mo (36–76)	Tubular	80% No repeat instrumentation
Bhargava et al,[95] 2008	5	Dermis	Buccal mucosa cells	34 mo (32–37)	Onlay	60%, Need for repeat urethroplasty
Ram-Liebig et al,[96] 2015	21	MukoCell	Oral mucosa cells	18 mo (13–22)	Ventral onlay	80.9%, Restricture requiring intervention

Abbreviations: ACMG, acellular matrix graft; Avg, average; F/U, follow-up; PGA, polyglycolic acid; SMCs, smooth muscle cells; UCs, urothelial cells.

tissue engineering for urethral reconstruction will certainly continue to expand; but as there have not yet been any clinical trials with these materials, large-scale implementation of this technology is likely still many years away.

Clinical Studies of Tissue-Engineered Grafts

A growing number of small studies of tissue-engineered urethral grafts in human subjects have been performed to date. The results of these studies are summarized in **Table 4**. Most of the procedures used acellular matrix grafts, either SIS[65,83–90] or acellular human bladder matrix,[91,92] whereas 2 studies used grafts seeded with urothelial cells[93,94] and 2 used TEBM.[95,96] Although most reports used a biological graft, one study used a cell-seeded synthetic PGA scaffold.[94] There exists considerable variability between studies, as well as within individual studies, regarding the technique for graft placement, including dorsal and ventral onlay, ventral inlay, tubularized urethral substitution, or endoscopic deployment of urethral grafts. Additionally, there is a range of patient cohort sizes, length of follow-up, and definition of success, making these studies difficult to directly compare. Across all studies, success ranged from 20% to 100%, but focusing on studies larger than 20 patients that have a minimum of 2 years follow-up finds a success rate of 76% to 100%.[85,88,89,92] The one clinical study of synthetic matrix graft reported 80% success in 5 patients,[94] which is comparable with the larger experience with biological grafts. Comparison of surgical techniques shows no clear superiority of any technique, with success varying even between studies using a similar approach and matrix material.

Most graft failures occurred within the first 6 months of implant. Graft reepithelialization was documented within the first 2 weeks and muscle fiber organization within 3 months following urethroplasty,[85] which is consistent with animal models of matrix reepithelialization.[67] This finding reinforces that the early postoperative phase is the critical time period for matrix graft uptake. Although failures have been reported as late as 18 months postoperatively,[89] the restricture rate generally drops off after 6 months. Besides stricture recurrence, the spectrum of postoperative complications following matrix urethroplasty is similar to that of native buccal mucosa grafts, including reports of urethrocutaneous fistula, postoperative incontinence, and erectile dysfunction.

Two studies have reported TEBM results in human subjects, one testing the commercial TEBM product MukoCell[96] and the other specifically evaluating patients with lichen sclerosus–induced

strictures.[95] Ram-Liebig and colleagues[96] reported the preliminary findings for their MukoCell off-the-shelf TEBM graft. At 18 months of follow-up they achieved an 80.9% success for 21 patients undergoing urethral reconstruction. This degree of success contrasts with the findings in the patients with lichen sclerosus, for which TEBM needed partial or complete revision in 2 of 5 patients and the remaining 3 were able to void but required DVIU or serial urethral dilations to maintain patency. These findings correlate with the high recurrence for lichen sclerosus in traditional urethral reconstruction techniques, with reports ranging from 20% to 50%.[97,98]

To compare tissue-engineered grafts with the current standard technique, el Kassaby and colleagues[91] randomized 30 total patients to undergo urethroplasty with acellular bladder mucosa graft (ABMG) versus native buccal mucosa graft. Success was defined as maintained voiding pattern postoperatively and no need for further intervention. All patient treated with buccal mucosa had successful outcomes, compared with 67% of patients treated with ABMG. Length, causes, or location of stricture did not influence outcomes. However, a possible role for ABMG is noted when patients are stratified by number of prior procedures. They reported 89% success (8 of 9) for patients with 0 to 1 prior procedures compared with 33% success (2 of 6) for patients with 2 or more prior procedures.

Although tissue-engineered grafts have a solid foundation in basic science and animal models, more clinical trials are needed to confirm their utility in humans. These grafts will have to prove their ability to overcome the challenges common to all grafts, including graft adhesion, contracture, and fibrosis. Initial clinical trials are promising, and more studies will help elucidate the best matrices and cellular material to achieve optimal urethral reconstruction results.

SUMMARY

Buccal mucosa grafts for urethral reconstruction have ushered in an era of durable grafts with well-documented success for urethral reconstruction. However, there are several circumstances whereby buccal mucosa is either inappropriate or inadequate to repair a given stricture. This situation has pushed reconstructive urologists to explore new approaches to stricture treatment, including new platforms for management or new sources of graft material. Endoscopic injection of antifibrotic agents is an interesting prospect for less invasive treatment of appropriately selected patients. A more extensive experience with these agents will be needed in order to clearly define their role within the current stricture treatment algorithm.

When performing augmentation urethroplasty, a reconstructive urologist should have multiple grafts at their disposal to fit the needs of a given patient. In addition to buccal mucosa, one should be comfortable with lingual mucosa and full-thickness skin grafts, although new autologous grafts, including colonic mucosa, may also become a standard in the armamentarium of a reconstructive surgeon. Tissue engineering opens an entirely new perspective on urethral grafts that would provide essentially unlimited graft material without the harvest-related morbidity. However, with minimal clinical data currently available, widespread use of these grafts remains a goal for the future.

REFERENCES

1. Pansadoro V, Emiliozzi P. Internal urethrotomy in the management of anterior urethral strictures: long-term follow-up. J Urol 1996;156(1):73–5.
2. Mangera A, Patterson JM, Chapple CR. A systematic review of graft augmentation urethroplasty techniques for the treatment of anterior urethral strictures. Eur Urol 2011;59(5):797–814.
3. Ferguson B, Gray SD, Thibeault S. Time and dose effects of mitomycin C on extracellular matrix fibroblasts and proteins. Laryngoscope 2005;115(1):110–5.
4. Ayyildiz A, Nuhoglu B, Gülerkaya B, et al. Effect of intraurethral mitomycin-C on healing and fibrosis in rats with experimentally induced urethral stricture. Int J Urol 2004;11(12):1122–6.
5. Ubell ML, Ettema SL, Toohill RJ, et al. Mitomycin-c application in airway stenosis surgery: analysis of safety and costs. Otolaryngol Head Neck Surg 2006;134(3):403–6.
6. Smith ME, Elstad M. Mitomycin C and the endoscopic treatment of laryngotracheal stenosis: are two applications better than one? Laryngoscope 2009;119(2):272–83.
7. Murakami M, Mori S, Kunitomo N. Studies on the pterygium. V. Follow-up information of mitomycin C treatment. Nippon Ganka Gakkai Zasshi 1967;71(4):351–8 [in Japanese].
8. Mueller CM, Beaunoyer M, St-Vil D. Topical mitomycin-C for the treatment of anal stricture. J Pediatr Surg 2010;45(1):241–4.
9. Dolmetsch AM. Nonlaser endoscopic endonasal dacryocystorhinostomy with adjunctive mitomycin C in nasolacrimal duct obstruction in adults. Ophthalmology 2010;117(5):1037–40.
10. Betalli P, De Corti F, Minucci D, et al. Successful topical treatment with mitomycin-C in a female with post-brachytherapy vaginal stricture. Pediatr Blood Cancer 2008;51(4):550–2.
11. Wolfram D, Tzankov A, Pulzl P, et al. Hypertrophic scars and keloids–a review of their pathophysiology, risk factors, and therapeutic management. Dermatol Surg 2009;35(2):171–81.
12. Poynter JH, Levy J. Balanitis xerotica obliterans: effective treatment with topical and sublesional corticosteroids. Br J Urol 1967;39(4):420–5.
13. Tavakkoli Tabassi K, Yarmohamadi A, Mohammadi S. Triamcinolone injection following internal urethrotomy for treatment of urethral stricture. Urol J 2011;8(2):132–6.
14. Mazdak H, Izadpanahi MH, Ghalamkari A, et al. Internal urethrotomy and intraurethral submucosal injection of triamcinolone in short bulbar urethral strictures. Int Urol Nephrol 2010;42(3):565–8.
15. Zhang K, Qi E, Zhang Y, et al. Efficacy and safety of local steroids for urethra strictures: a systematic review and meta-analysis. J Endourol 2014;28(8):962–8.
16. Mazdak H, Meshki I, Ghassami F. Effect of mitomycin C on anterior urethral stricture recurrence after internal urethrotomy. Eur Urol 2007;51(4):1089–92 [discussion: 1092].
17. Ali L, Shahzad M, Orakzai N, et al. Efficacy of mitomycin C in reducing recurrence of anterior urethral stricture after internal optical urethrotomy. Korean J Urol 2015;56(9):650–5.
18. Cevik M, Demir T, Karadag CA, et al. Preliminary study of efficacy of hyaluronic acid on caustic esophageal burns in an experimental rat model. J Pediatr Surg 2013;48(4):716–23.
19. Chung JH, Kang DH, Choi HY, et al. The effects of hyaluronic acid and carboxymethylcellulose in preventing recurrence of urethral stricture after endoscopic internal urethrotomy: a multicenter, randomized controlled, single-blinded study. J Endourol 2013;27(6):756–62.
20. Kumar S, Garg N, Singh SK, et al. Efficacy of optical internal urethrotomy and intralesional injection of Vatsala-Santosh PGI tri-inject (triamcinolone, mitomycin C, and hyaluronidase) in the treatment of anterior urethral stricture. Adv Urol 2014;2014:192710.
21. Khera M, Boone TB, Smith CP. Botulinum toxin type A: a novel approach to the treatment of recurrent urethral strictures. J Urol 2004;172(2):574–5.
22. Sangkum P, Yafi FA, Kim H, et al. Collagenase clostridium histolyticum (Xiaflex) for the treatment of urethral stricture disease in a rat model of urethral fibrosis. Urology 2015;86(3):647.e1-6.
23. Uyeturk U, Gucuk A, Firat T, et al. Effect of mitomycin, bevacizumab, and 5-fluorouracil to inhibit urethral fibrosis in a rabbit model. J Endourol 2014;28(11):1363–7.
24. Jaidane M, Ali-El-Dein B, Ounaies A, et al. The use of halofuginone in limiting urethral stricture formation

and recurrence: an experimental study in rabbits. J Urol 2003;170(5):2049–52.

25. Presman D, Greenfield DL. Reconstruction of the perineal urethra with a free full-thickness skin graft from the prepuce. J Urol 1953;69(5):677–80.

26. Devine CJ, Horton CE. A one stage hypospadias repair. J Urol 1961;85:166–72.

27. Wessells H, McAninch JW. Current controversies in anterior urethral stricture repair: free-graft versus pedicled skin-flap reconstruction. World J Urol 1998;16(3):175–80.

28. Dubey D, Vijjan V, Kapoor R, et al. Dorsal onlay buccal mucosa versus penile skin flap urethroplasty for anterior urethral strictures: results from a randomized prospective trial. J Urol 2007;178(6):2466–9.

29. Greenwell TJ, Venn SN, Mundy AR. Changing practice in anterior urethroplasty. BJU Int 1999;83(6):631–5.

30. Dubey D, Kumar A, Bansal P, et al. Substitution urethroplasty for anterior urethral strictures: a critical appraisal of various techniques. BJU Int 2003;91(3):215–8.

31. Lumen N, Oosterlinck W, Hoebeke P. Urethral reconstruction using buccal mucosa or penile skin grafts: systematic review and meta-analysis. Urol Int 2012;89(4):387–94.

32. Barbagli G, Kulkarni SB, Fossati N, et al. Long-term follow-up and deterioration rate of anterior substitution urethroplasty. J Urol 2014;192(3):808–13.

33. Manoj B, Sanjeev N, Pandurang PN, et al. Postauricular skin as an alternative to oral mucosa for anterior onlay graft urethroplasty: a preliminary experience in patients with oral mucosa changes. Urology 2009;74(2):345–8.

34. Nitkunan T, Johal N, O'Malley K, et al. Secondary hypospadias repair in two stages. J Pediatr Urol 2006;2(6):559–63.

35. Chen ML, Odom BD, Johnson LJ, et al. Combining ventral buccal mucosal graft onlay and dorsal full thickness skin graft inlay decreases failure rates in long bulbar strictures (>/=6 cm). Urology 2013;81(4):899–902.

36. Liu JS, Han J, Said M, et al. Long-term outcomes of urethroplasty with abdominal wall skin grafts. Urology 2015;85(1):258–62.

37. Schreiter F, Noll F. Mesh graft urethroplasty using split thickness skin graft or foreskin. J Urol 1989;142(5):1223–6.

38. Kessler TM, Schreiter F, Kralidis G, et al. Long-term results of surgery for urethral stricture: a statistical analysis. J Urol 2003;170(3):840–4.

39. Pfalzgraf D, Olianas R, Schreiter F, et al. Two-staged urethroplasty: buccal mucosa and mesh graft techniques. Aktuelle Urol 2010;41(Suppl 1):S5–9.

40. Palminteri E, Brandes SB, Djordjevic M. Urethral reconstruction in lichen sclerosus. Curr Opin Urol 2012;22(6):478–83.

41. Dubey D, Sehgal A, Srivastava A, et al. Buccal mucosal urethroplasty for balanitis xerotica obliterans related urethral strictures: the outcome of 1 and 2-stage techniques. J Urol 2005;173(2):463–6.

42. Simonato A, Gregori A, Ambruosi C, et al. Lingual mucosal graft urethroplasty for anterior urethral reconstruction. Eur Urol 2008;54(1):79–85.

43. Barbagli G, De Angelis M, Romano G, et al. The use of lingual mucosal graft in adult anterior urethroplasty: surgical steps and short-term outcome. Eur Urol 2008;54(3):671–6.

44. Xu YM, Fu Q, Sa YL, et al. Treatment of urethral strictures using lingual mucosas urethroplasty: experience of 92 cases. Chin Med J 2010;123(4):458–62.

45. Das SK, Kumar A, Sharma GK, et al. Lingual mucosal graft urethroplasty for anterior urethral strictures. Urology 2009;73(1):105–8.

46. Sharma GK, Pandey A, Bansal H, et al. Dorsal onlay lingual mucosal graft urethroplasty for urethral strictures in women. BJU Int 2010;105(9):1309–12.

47. Abdelhameed H, Elgamal S, Farha MA, et al. The long-term results of lingual mucosal grafts for repairing long anterior urethral strictures. Arab J Urol 2015;13(2):128–33.

48. Li HB, Xu YM, Fu Q, et al. One-stage dorsal lingual mucosal graft urethroplasty for the treatment of failed hypospadias repair. Asian J Androl 2016;18(3):467–70.

49. Sharma AK, Chandrashekar R, Keshavamurthy R, et al. Lingual versus buccal mucosa graft urethroplasty for anterior urethral stricture: a prospective comparative analysis. Int J Urol 2013;20(12):1199–203.

50. Chauhan S, Yadav SS, Tomar V. Outcome of buccal mucosa and lingual mucosa graft urethroplasty in the management of urethral strictures: a comparative study. Urol Ann 2016;8(1):36–41.

51. Lumen N, Vierstraete-Verlinde S, Oosterlinck W, et al. Buccal versus lingual mucosa graft in anterior urethroplasty: a prospective comparison of surgical outcome and donor site morbidity. J Urol 2016;195(1):112–7.

52. Maarouf AM, Elsayed ER, Ragab A, et al. Buccal versus lingual mucosal graft urethroplasty for complex hypospadias repair. J Pediatr Urol 2013;9(6 Pt A):754–8.

53. Xu YM, Feng C, Sa YL, et al. Outcome of 1-stage urethroplasty using oral mucosal grafts for the treatment of urethral strictures associated with genital lichen sclerosus. Urology 2014;83(1):232–6.

54. Simonato A, Gregori A. Oral complications after lingual mucosal graft harvest for urethroplasty. ANZ J Surg 2008;78(10):933–4.

55. Kumar A, Goyal NK, Das SK, et al. Oral complications after lingual mucosal graft harvest for urethroplasty. ANZ J Surg 2007;77(11):970–3.

56. Kinkead TM, Borzi PA, Duffy PG, et al. Long-term follow-up of bladder mucosa graft for male urethral reconstruction. J Urol 1994;151(4):1056–8.

57. Xu YM, Qiao Y, Sa YL, et al. 1-stage urethral reconstruction using colonic mucosa graft for the treatment of a long complex urethral stricture. J Urol 2004;171(1):220–3 [discussion: 223].

58. Xu YM, Qiao Y, Sa YL, et al. Urethral reconstruction using colonic mucosa graft for complex strictures. J Urol 2009;182(3):1040–3.

59. Palmer DA, Marcello PW, Zinman LN, et al. Urethral reconstruction with rectal mucosa graft onlay: a novel, minimally invasive technique. J Urol 2016; 196(3):782–6.

60. Nagele U, Maurer S, Feil G, et al. In vitro investigations of tissue-engineered multilayered urothelium established from bladder washings. Eur Urol 2008; 54(6):1414–22.

61. de Kemp V, de Graaf P, Fledderus JO, et al. Tissue engineering for human urethral reconstruction: systematic review of recent literature. PLoS One 2015; 10(2):e0118653.

62. Lovett ML, Cannizzaro CM, Vunjak-Novakovic G, et al. Gel spinning of silk tubes for tissue engineering. Biomaterials 2008;29(35):4650–7.

63. Wünsch L, Ehlers EM, Russlies M. Matrix testing for urothelial tissue engineering. Eur J Pediatr Surg 2005;15(3):164–9.

64. Dorin RP, Pohl HG, De Filippo RE, et al. Tubularized urethral replacement with unseeded matrices: what is the maximum distance for normal tissue regeneration? World J Urol 2008;26(4):323–6.

65. le Roux PJ. Endoscopic urethroplasty with unseeded small intestinal submucosa collagen matrix grafts: a pilot study. J Urol 2005;173(1):140–3.

66. De Filippo RE, Yoo JJ, Atala A. Urethral replacement using cell seeded tubularized collagen matrices. J Urol 2002;168(4 Pt 2):1789–92 [discussion: 1792–3].

67. De Filippo RE, Kornitzer BS, Yoo JJ, et al. Penile urethra replacement with autologous cell-seeded tubularized collagen matrices. J Tissue Eng Regen Med 2015;9(3):257–64.

68. Hudson AE, Carmean N, Bassuk JA. Extracellular matrix protein coatings for facilitation of urothelial cell attachment. Tissue Eng 2007;13(9):2219–25.

69. Ye Q, Zund G, Jockenhoevel S, et al. Scaffold precoating with human autologous extracellular matrix for improved cell attachment in cardiovascular tissue engineering. ASAIO J 2000;46(6):730–3.

70. Uchida N, Sivaraman S, Amoroso NJ, et al. Nanometer-sized extracellular matrix coating on polymer-based scaffold for tissue engineering applications. J Biomed Mater Res A 2016;104(1): 94–103.

71. Bisson I, Hilborn J, Wurm F, et al. Human urothelial cells grown on collagen adsorbed to surface-modified polymers. Urology 2002;60(1):176–80.

72. Kundu AK, Gelman J, Tyson DR. Composite thin film and electrospun biomaterials for urologic tissue reconstruction. Biotechnol Bioeng 2011;108(1): 207–15.

73. Kimuli M, Eardley I, Southgate J. In vitro assessment of decellularized porcine dermis as a matrix for urinary tract reconstruction. BJU Int 2004;94(6): 859–66.

74. Zhang Y, Kropp BP, Moore P, et al. Coculture of bladder urothelial and smooth muscle cells on small intestinal submucosa: potential applications for tissue engineering technology. J Urol 2000;164(3 Pt 2):928–34 [discussion: 934–5].

75. Orabi H, Rousseau A, Laterreur V, et al. Optimization of the current self-assembled urinary bladder model: organ-specific stroma and smooth muscle inclusion. Can Urol Assoc J 2015;9(9–10):E599–607.

76. Bhargava S, Chapple CR, Bullock AJ, et al. Tissue-engineered buccal mucosa for substitution urethroplasty. BJU Int 2004;93(6):807–11.

77. Chung YG, Tu D, Franck D, et al. Acellular bi-layer silk fibroin scaffolds support tissue regeneration in a rabbit model of onlay urethroplasty. PLoS One 2014;9(3):e91592.

78. Frimberger D, Morales N, Shamblott M, et al. Human embryoid body-derived stem cells in bladder regeneration using rodent model. Urology 2005;65(4): 827–32.

79. Li CL, Liao WB, Yang SX, et al. Urethral reconstruction using bone marrow mesenchymal stem cell- and smooth muscle cell-seeded bladder acellular matrix. Transplant Proc 2013;45(9):3402–7.

80. Wu S, Liu Y, Bharadwaj S, et al. Human urine-derived stem cells seeded in a modified 3D porous small intestinal submucosa scaffold for urethral tissue engineering. Biomaterials 2011;32(5):1317–26.

81. Li H, Xu Y, Xie H, et al. Epithelial-differentiated adipose-derived stem cells seeded bladder acellular matrix grafts for urethral reconstruction: an animal model. Tissue Eng Part A 2014;20(3–4):774–84.

82. Fu Q, Cao YL. Tissue engineering and stem cell application of urethroplasty: from bench to bedside. Urology 2012;79(2):246–53.

83. Donkov II, Bashir A, Elenkov CH, et al. Dorsal onlay augmentation urethroplasty with small intestinal submucosa: modified Barbagli technique for strictures of the bulbar urethra. Int J Urol 2006;13(11):1415–7.

84. Hauser S, Bastian PJ, Fechner G, et al. Small intestine submucosa in urethral stricture repair in a consecutive series. Urology 2006;68(2):263–6.

85. Fiala R, Vidlar A, Vrtal R, et al. Porcine small intestinal submucosa graft for repair of anterior urethral strictures. Eur Urol 2007;51(6):1702–8 [discussion: 1708].

86. Farahat YA, Elbahnasy AM, El-Gamal OM, et al. Endoscopic urethroplasty using small intestinal submucosal patch in cases of recurrent urethral stricture: a preliminary study. J Endourol 2009;23(12): 2001–5.

87. Mantovani F, Trinchieri A, Mangiarotti B, et al. Reconstructive urethroplasty using porcine acellular matrix: preliminary results. Arch Ital Urol Androl 2002; 74(3):127–8 [in Italian].

88. Mantovani F, Tondelli E, Cozzi G, et al. Reconstructive urethroplasty using porcine acellular matrix (SIS): evolution of the grafting technique and results of 10-year experience. Urologia 2011;78(2):92–7 [in Italian].

89. Palminteri E, Berdondini E, Fusco F, et al. Long-term results of small intestinal submucosa graft in bulbar urethral reconstruction. Urology 2012;79(3): 695–701.

90. Orabi H, Safwat AS, Shahat A, et al. The use of small intestinal submucosa graft for hypospadias repair: pilot study. Arab J Urol 2013;11(4):415–20.

91. el-Kassaby A, AbouShwareb T, Atala A. Randomized comparative study between buccal mucosal and acellular bladder matrix grafts in complex anterior urethral strictures. J Urol 2008;179(4):1432–6.

92. el-Kassaby AW, Retik AB, Yoo JJ, et al. Urethral stricture repair with an off-the-shelf collagen matrix. J Urol 2003;169(1):170–3 [discussion: 173].

93. Fossum M, Skikuniene J, Orrego A, et al. Prepubertal follow-up after hypospadias repair with autologous in vitro cultured urothelial cells. Acta Paediatr 2012;101(7):755–60.

94. Raya-Rivera A, Esquiliano DR, Yoo JJ, et al. Tissue-engineered autologous urethras for patients who need reconstruction: an observational study. Lancet 2011;377(9772):1175–82.

95. Bhargava S, Patterson JM, Inman RD, et al. Tissue-engineered buccal mucosa urethroplasty-clinical outcomes. Eur Urol 2008;53(6):1263–9.

96. Ram-Liebig G, Bednarz J, Stuerzebecher B, et al. Regulatory challenges for autologous tissue engineered products on their way from bench to bedside in Europe. Adv Drug Deliv Rev 2015;82-83:181–91.

97. Erickson BA, Elliott SP, Myers JB, et al. Understanding the relationship between chronic systemic disease and lichen sclerosus urethral strictures. J Urol 2016;195(2):363–8.

98. Patel CK, Buckley JC, Zinman LN, et al. Outcomes for management of lichen sclerosus urethral strictures by 3 different techniques. Urology 2016;91: 215–21.

Index

Note: Page numbers of article titles are in **boldface** type.

Urol Clin N Am 44 (2017) 141–145
http://dx.doi.org/10.1016/S0094-0143(16)30110-0
0094-0143/17